Praise for *The Self-Health Revolution*

"We live in a country where financially motivated 'forces' cleverly assist you to become the unhealthiest version of yourself possible. If you care about your Self-Health, you owe it to your body to read *The Self-Health Revolution*. From the pharmaceutical to farming industries, from Coca-Cola to cows, J. Michael Zenn reveals truths you need to know to outwit those forces and to become the healthiest and happiest 'you' you have ever known. I share the Self-Health Smoothie recipe with all patients who ask, 'What can I do to reduce my chances of getting cancer?' and I tell them to make extra for their husbands and children, too. I'm pretty sure my three toddlers will be impervious to countless ailments by age ten!"

—**Kristi Funk, MD, FACS,** breast cancer surgeon

"I think this book is great! Michael Zenn's *The Self-Health Revolution* is a very practical guide for anybody interested in improving their health and their lives. I am encouraging everyone to read this book. If ever there was a right message, at the right time, this is it."

—**David T. Feinberg, MD, MBA,**
president of UCLA Health System, and vice chancellor
and CEO of UCLA Hospital System

"From the moment I picked the book up, I was hooked. I've never endorsed a book, but this is one of the best books on health and wellness I have ever read. Finally, someone has written a book that is so simple-to-read, easy-to-understand and just makes plain sense. I was shocked and delighted to discover, "We are what we eat . . . eats!" and so many other life-changing revelations. Michael Zenn wisely points out that health is not just about what you're eating but also 'what's eating you.' The chapters on gratitude and happiness left me inspired and challenged. Everyone owes it to themself to read this book!"

—**Jeffrey Nagel,** CEO of Nature's Bounty / Vitamin World,
one of the world's largest vitamins,
minerals, and supplements companies

"What a masterful and inspired job of bringing together a mountain of life-saving information into one blazing page-turner. If ever there was a single book anyone interested in his or her health and well-being should read without fail, this is it! This groundbreaking, commonsense, eye-opening read will show you the hidden reasons why so many people are getting sicker, growing fatter, feeling older than their years, and dying younger than they should. J. Michael Zenn will show you how you can quickly take control of your own Self-Health and determine your own health destiny. Are you as fit as you wish to be? Do you have the energy you desire? Are you free from pain, ill health, and disease? Are you aging faster than you would like? Discover how you can directly determine how long and how well you will live. Michael and I share many similarities on our healing journeys. He too began to study nutrition as a means to overcome serious health problems that baffled the medical community. Let Michael show you the powerful evidence that will convince any common sense person that our Self-Health destiny is totally within our grasp. Read this book now, put it into practice, and share it with the people you love. You will be glad for the rest of your long and healthy life."

—**Harvey Diamond,** author of *Fit for Life*

"What has happened to our food today? Now, finally, a book that clearly exposes the causes of our massive health problems! *The Self-Health Revolution* is a simple, easy-to-follow guide to optimum health."

—**Tom Campanaro,** founder and CEO of Total Gym

"J. Michael Zenn has written a wonderful book on health that accurately describes the growing health problems in America. He provides invaluable suggestions which can help anyone to lose weight and live a life full of vitality and superb health. Obesity, diabetes, heart disease, stroke, and cancer are primarily lifestyle diseases that we need not ever suffer from, but which currently result from the unhealthy diets and lifestyles that most Americans indulge in. What we need to do is to wholeheartedly embrace the principles of healthy eating and healthy living outlined in *The Self-Health Revolution*. I enthusiastically recommend this book!"

—**John Mackey,** co-founder and co-CEO of Whole Foods Market

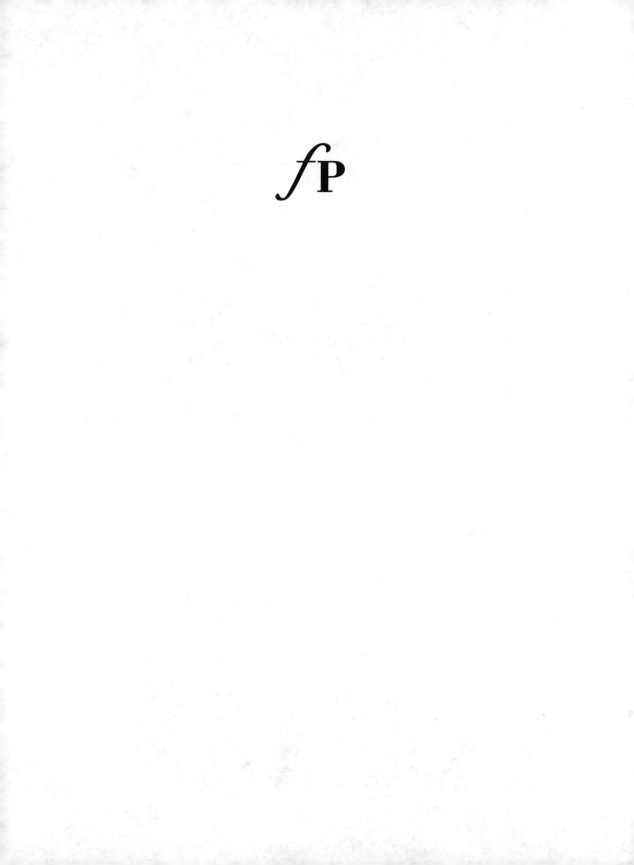

You must take personal responsibility for your life.
You cannot change the circumstances, the seasons,
or the wind, but you can change yourself.
—Jim Rohn, America's foremost business philosopher

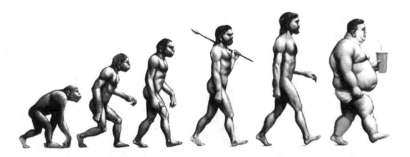

THE
SELF
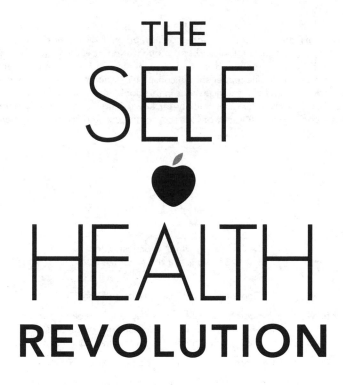
HEALTH
REVOLUTION

J. Michael Zenn

FREE PRESS

New York   London   Toronto   Sydney   New Delhi

NOTE TO READERS

Free Press
A Division of Simon & Schuster, Inc.
1230 Avenue of the Americas
New York, NY 10020

First Free Press trade paperback edition November 2012

FREE PRESS and colophon are trademarks of Simon & Schuster, Inc.

For information about special discounts for bulk purchases, please contact Simon & Schuster Special Sales at 1-866-506-1949 or business@simonandschuster.com.

The Simon & Schuster Speakers Bureau can bring authors to your live event. For more information or to book an event, contact the Simon & Schuster Speakers Bureau at 1-866-248-3049 or visit our website at www.simonspeakers.com.

Manufactured in the United States of America

1 3 5 7 9 10 8 6 4 2

Library of Congress Cataloging-in-Publication Data

Zenn, J. Michael.
The self-health revolution / J. Michael Zenn.
    p. cm.
Summary: "How to take charge of your health by cutting out toxins and eating healthful foods"—Provided by publisher.
Includes bibliographical references.
1. Health. 2. Nutrition. 3. Physical fitness. 4. Self-care, Health. I. Title.
RA776.Z46 2012
613—dc23
2012023321
ISBN 978-1-4767-0359-6
ISBN 978-1-4767-0400-5 (ebook)

Read This Before Anything Else!

First of all, let me personally thank you for taking the time to read this book. I realize you are busy and there are many things in your life begging for your attention. By purchasing this book, you are demonstrating how committed you are to seeking information that will improve your life and the lives of those you love.

If the statistics are accurate, 50 percent of those who begin to read this book will not finish; 25 percent will not read beyond the second chapter. In order for you to benefit fully from this book, I am going to ask you to make a decision right now to read the entire book. **Start at the beginning and read this book from cover to cover. Please do not jump ahead or jump around looking for an immediate answer to your questions.** I know you will be tempted to do so, but please be patient and follow this advice. All the information in this book is put together in a specific order for a reason. *The Self-Health Revolution* will not make sense to you if you read parts out of their intended context.

You may notice that many concepts are repeated throughout this book. This is done by design. I believe in the rule of five: *Most of us need to hear something five times before we clearly understand it.* The rule of five certainly applies to me, and I hope it will help you to understand and digest the foundational principles of Self-Health.

In the first half of this book you will be exposed to some shocking and disturbing information. You may feel a little overwhelmed at times. These data are painful to read but necessary to know. I ask you to please hang in there because the second half of the book will give you clear, simple, and actionable responses to these negative realities.

Throughout this book you may read about companies, organizations, products, and other thought leaders that I truly believe in and even endorse. *I do not receive money from any of these companies (including Whole Foods Market) for the mentions in this book, and I include only the ones that I have personally tested and wholeheartedly believe in.* I would never put profits above principles, and certainly not before the people I am desperately trying to help by writing this book.

You might be thinking, *Who is this guy to write a book about Self-Health? Why should I listen to him? What are his credentials?* My credentials are simple. I am an average, ordinary person who has discovered an extraordinary secret that has dramatically changed my health and the health of countless others. This life-changing information does not originate with me. Its authority is not validated by my pedigree or my personal genius (thank God). I am simply someone who has taken the time and effort to read over a hundred books on the subject, study a thousand websites, and listen to countless videos, CDs, and tapes. I've made calls to experts all over the country and traveled hundreds of miles to talk with some of the smartest people I could find in order to fuel my own Self-Health Revolution. In this book I am sharing what has powerfully worked for me. **The power of *The Self-Health Revolution* is found in the message, not the messenger.**

For those of you who are a little skeptical, as I was when I first heard some of these facts, there are sources listed at the end of this book to back up the stunning statistics and data presented. I challenge you to research anything you find in this book to confirm whether it's true. But please don't give in to your disbelief and doubt and simply close the pages of this book and deny its claims without any investigation. *The Self-Health Revolution* makes some riveting and audacious claims. If these claims are false, then this book will take its place on history's garbage heap of misleading and useless health books. *But if these claims prove to be true, then they have astronomical implications for your health and the health of everyone that you care about.*

So do yourself the service of reading this book page after page, from cover to cover. Don't be part of the 50 percent who miss out and don't discover what Self-Health is all about. Keep your skepticism intact, test everything, but proceed with an open mind. Please wait until you've read—and thought about—the whole book before you form your final opinions regarding the Self-Health Revolution. If you do, you may be surprised and delighted with the results of your due diligence.

Please contact me with your comments, questions, ideas, and testimonials.

JMichaelZenn@gmail.com

THE
SELF
HEALTH
REVOLUTION

*There is one thing stronger than all the armies of the world
and that is an idea whose time has come.*
—Victor Hugo

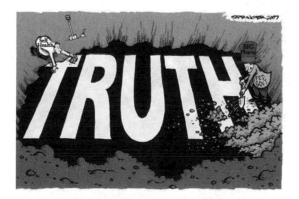

Acknowledgments

I dedicate this book to my personal hero, my dad, who truly demonstrated the meaning of love; to my mom, who encouraged me to see the beauty and genius of nature; to my children, Jonathan and Amber, who daily make me glad and proud to be a father.

This book has been the culmination of my entire life's victories and failures, pains and pleasures. I have met so many influential people who have fatefully crossed my path and unselfishly shared invaluable gifts of wisdom and belief. It is impossible to name them all, but I would like to applaud a few.

I express my deepest gratitude to the incredibly capable Simon & Schuster publishing team: Including Suzanne Donahue, V.P., Associate Publisher; Leslie Meredith, V.P., Senior Editor; Dominick Anfuso, V.P., Senior Editor; Donna Loffredo, Associate Editor; Carisa Hays, V.P., Director of Publicity; Larry Hughes, Associate Director of Publicity; Kristin Matzen, Associate Publicist; Nicole Judge, Director of Marketing; Claire Kelley, Marketing Manager; Phil Metcalf, Production Editor; Erich Hobbing, Interior Designer; Eric Fuentecilla, Jacket Designer; and of course the amazingly talented Martha Levin, Executive Vice President and Publisher, without whom this project would not have been done.

This sterling Free Press team not only worked incredibly hard on this book but also showed how deeply they believe in its message, purpose, and passion. It's easy to see why they are one of the most successful publishing teams in the history of the industry.

I would also like to thank my publicist, Stephen Hanselman, who believed in this project from day one. Stephen is truly one of the very best agents in the world and represents a who's who of A-list authors. His knowledge of the publishing world is unsurpassed.

I would like to give special thanks to Deborah Morin and John Mackey, who have demonstrated, as much or more than any two people on Earth, a deep commitment to educating our country about the dire need for self-health and providing a wonderful place for people to find it. They are and always will be, my heroes.

To my good friend Libby, an angel sent from the heavens to rescue me. You lifted me up, raised my arms, and helped me stand again. I am forever in your debt.

Most important, I want to thank the One who created me and made me for such a time as this. My life is nothing but a gift given by this magnificent being whom I love and adore.

Finally, I would like to thank Harvey Diamond, the author of *Fit for Life*, a book that was #1 on the *New York Times* bestseller list an unprecedented forty consecutive weeks and that has become one of the top twenty-five bestselling books in publishing history, taking its place alongside the likes of *Gone with the Wind* and the Bible. Harvey has been a great inspiration and mentor, and I owe many of the beliefs in this book to his compassionate genius.

Contents

*Did you know that right now,
during this massive financial downturn,
you are three times more likely to get sick?*

Not since 1929 have we seen such financial fear, stress, and panic. What may be churning toward us now is what many are calling the "perfect storm" or, even worse, "financial Armageddon." Yet whether or not you believe the wholesale hype, if a deeper or even a double-dip recession materializes, the biggest risk may not be to your wallet, 401(k), life savings, or bank account.

A shocking new report shows that the most damaging impact of a financial crisis is to your own personal health. In a study of 1,800 people, 91 percent experienced declining health when exposed to financial stress. They were actually three times more likely to get sick—three times more readily diagnosed with seasonal illnesses, chronic disease, high blood pressure, high cholesterol, heart disease, cancer, depression, and other stress-related diseases—than people whose lives were financially stable.

In the Great Depression, malnutrition and chronic illness more than tripled. In times of financial hardship, worries abound, and we all know that stress dramatically lowers the ability of the immune system to fight infection. Focused on fear, people tend to indulge in cheaper, comfort foods (toxins), exercise routines are reduced (reducing oxygen in the blood), and more expensive, nutrient-rich foods, probiotics, and supplements are set aside (resulting in malnutrition). Whatever the approaching storm may bring, you must decide now not to join the ranks of the thousands of American victims that are surely caught up in this Self-Health–destructive tsunami.

Join the Self-Health Revolution now! Plan at this moment to protect your and your family's health from the current crisis. Commit personally to the ten-day challenge in this book. If it works, make it part of your lifestyle and belief system forever. Then you won't have to worry about sickness-inducing financial storms. It has certainly worked for me. I haven't been sick (not even a cold) in years!

What We Don't Know Is That We **Don't Know**

*It's not so much what folks don't know that
causes problems. It's what they do know that ain't so.*
—Artemus Ward, American humorist

We didn't know. I know that *I* didn't know. And I'm pretty darn sure that *they* didn't want us to know.

For some time now, Americans have been comfortable with the notion that doctors, the medical profession, the pharmaceutical industry, big food companies, and even the folks at the U.S. Food and Drug Administration would do the worrying about our nutrition and health for us. We are in for a big surprise. If Hurricane Katrina, the Gulf oil spill, and the massive federal deficit reveal anything about our government's ability to anticipate and fix our problems, it's the fact that our huge government and institutions are not our saviors and are capable of almost incomprehensible mistakes and ignorance.

Could the government be equally as wrong about what we eat and how it affects our health? We may think that any food that carries the federal government's stamp of approval is healthful. Can we really trust it? It seems that since our bellies are full and we eat what the giant food companies, advertisers, and government officials say we should eat, we must be getting all the nutrients we need to be healthy. But how can we be certain?

Many of us thought it was okay to eat what everybody else ate just because everybody else was eating it.

Now we know that if we do, we may end up with all the diseases that everybody else is getting (in greater and greater numbers).

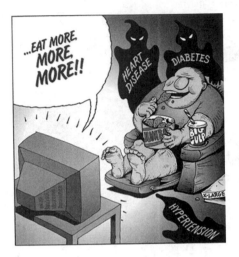

The "Giant Wings Conspiracy"

Likewise, some folks think the pharmaceutical companies toil 24/7 to bring us fountains of youth in the form of Little Purple Pills. But perhaps the drug companies have a deeper motivation. These companies mostly make money from sick people, not dead people— not healthy people but sick people, those stuck somewhere between health and death, destined to live life struggling with a chronic illness, popping a chronic pill. So drug companies may not be overly concerned about the long-term effects of what you're eating, even if it's something bad for you, because, in the end, it gives them a few more customers.

You've heard of right-wing and left-wing conspiracies. Although this is *not* a conspiracy theory book, I do believe that there is today what some might consider a "Giant Wings Conspiracy." It was conceived to make you eat the wrong things, live with uncured diseases, take unnecessary drugs, and remain chronically ill on these drugs for the rest of your life. The medical institutions, the food companies, and the pharmaceutical industry make a lot of money from sick people. Is it possible they *want* us to be sick? Could they really be that corrupt, grossly inept, or simply indifferent?

The Love of Money

I know this description may seem a little extreme. Let me make it clear that I do not believe there is anything wrong with business owners, executives, or corporations making lots of money if they provide a great service or product that actually helps people. In that same spirit, I hope this book is successful. But companies that make money by taking advantage of the ignorance of their customers, although they have the legal right to exist, also deserve to be exposed. Is it possible that all these huge companies and organizations employing thousands of people are somehow conspiring against us? I don't think it's necessarily personal, nor do I believe it originates from most of the millions of rank-and-file employees within these companies. I am sure many of these organizations started on the path that has led them to where they are today with the very best of intentions. Could it be that something happened to the officials and shareholders of these organizations that ultimately led them to be driven by another motivation altogether?

Unfortunately, I don't even have to say it, do I? It's a story that's been told in every generation. It's the story of how good people under pressure unintentionally become greedy and eventually are willing to say anything, do anything, and take advantage of anyone in order to make more money. As the Bible says, "The love of money is the root of all evil." Would you really be surprised to find out that greed is such a powerful force in the world today?

No One Loves You Like You Do

My point is not to bash these organizations or companies, although they should be exposed. I want to prove to you that no one will take care of you as well as you can. Here's something you can take to the bank: No one loves you like you do. When it comes to saving your own life, protecting your and your family's health from the onslaught of the greedy companies and organizations that will sell you anything, feed you anything, inject you with any-

thing, it's time to seize your own Self-Health. It may be just the right time to take back what's yours and stop entrusting something so valuable and so precious to anyone else. It's something only you can do and something you must be willing to do. If you don't do it, there are certainly those who are all too happy to take control of your Self-Health for you.

That's why I wrote this book: to help myself and to help you. I want to share with you what I've learned. I want to share how just three simple steps can change your life. You'll be able to experience a personal Self-Health Revolution! You'll wake up energized, lose more weight, improve your digestion, have better bathroom experiences, get rid of many aches and pains, equip your body to fight off seasonal and chronic or fatal illness, sleep more deeply and soundly, increase sexual desire, and enjoy life as you've never enjoyed it before. Many people don't know what they are missing because they do not know how good it can be—how good life and health are truly meant to be.

Too Good to Be True?

I know this may sound too good to be true, unrealistic or even unbelievable. You might be thinking, *Now who's the one telling us anything we want to hear?* Fair enough. I can understand how you might feel, but please give me a chance to explain. What if there is actually something to this? Would you want to know more?

What I have discovered is not a new product, a new idea, a new fad diet, a network marketing scheme, a secret ingredient, or undiscovered truth. What I have uncovered and rediscovered are ancient truths—truths that come from the infinite wisdom of the universe, given by the Creator itself, passed down from generation to generation but forgotten by most of us in the modern world. It is truth that your great-great-grandmother may have known very well. It's a teaching practiced by civilizations throughout the ages, in remote regions of the world today, and perhaps even secretly adhered to in the households of a few modern Americans. It's a secret that has changed millions of lives through the ages and can powerfully change your life and the lives of those you love.

The Common Sense Corner

The secrets of Self-Health are truly simple and easy to understand. They will not cost you a fortune to put into practice; they won't demand hours and hours of your time; and they won't require you to commit to Herculean tasks or starvation diets or even radically change your current lifestyle. Self-Health will not request that you check your brains at the door and embrace some mystical teaching that contradicts common sense. Self-Health will strongly appeal to your intuition and logic. It will make sense to you because it indeed makes perfect sense. It is like something that you already know, something that you have simply forgotten because it has been so long since we have conjured this innate knowledge out of the cobwebs.

The Die in Dieting

I love food and love to eat. How about you? Eating is simply the most satisfying part of my day. I am not sure if there is anything else that I enjoy more than sitting down at a table that's covered in delicious food. Self-Health will not ask you to give up great food. We know diets don't work. Many have suffered and even died from being on the wrong diet. Diets are designed to

Facts do not cease to exist because they are ignored.
—ALDOUS HUXLEY,
VISIONARY WRITER

starve the body, but Self-Health will teach you how to feed the body by eating great food and lots of it. This is certainly not the teaching of an ascetic monk or a modern-day Buddha who wants to live life on a single bean a day. You will be able to eat more and better-tasting food and as much as you want. These are foods and flavors that are an experience beyond anything that you may have ever known—simply the best-tasting foods on the planet.

Again, I realize this all may sound like a fairy tale, but I assure you it is not. It is as real as the paper this ink is printed on. I know because I experienced it myself. I can write these words with all of the authority, integrity, and truthfulness in the world because Self-Health is something I have lived. It has changed my life forever, and I am totally committed to sharing this truth with as many people as possible for the rest of my life.

I know you are skeptical, and you should be. I want to help you become even more skeptical of the things you are told by those who have only one motive in mind: to separate you from your hard-earned money. I ask you to put me to the test. See if what I am saying is true. Try the Self-Health truths in this book and see if you don't get the same results I did. To use a food cliché, the proof is in the pudding. So taste the pudding, and if you do, I don't have one ounce of doubt about what you will discover.

Be Skeptical but Teachable

There is a difference between being close-minded and being skeptical. Some people don't want to know what they don't know. Among other things, this mind-set has been called the "head buried in the sand syndrome." Some people challenge the validity of uncomfortable information simply out of fear of having to change once they know the truth. So they decide that they would rather not know it at all. I understand this resistance, as I lived most of my life that way. However, such a mind-set can be dangerous. For example, I may not believe in the law of gravity, and I may even deny its existence, but that

Believe nothing, no matter where you read it or who said it, even if I have said it, unless it agrees with your own reason and your own common sense.

—BUDDHA

does not change the reality of gravity. If I were to fall or jump off a building, gravity would show that it truly is a law of the universe (whether or not I believe it).

The important question is not if you are skeptical, but if you are teachable. Are you open to believing in something and making changes once it has been proven to you that it is true? If so, then you are a learner and teachable. The noted scholar W. S. Howell says we pass through four distinct stages as we learn:

1. *Unconscious Incompetence:* You don't know what you don't know.

2. *Conscious Incompetence:* You discover you aren't as competent as you thought you were.

3. *Conscious Competence:* You begin serious efforts to progress and learn.

4. *Unconscious Competence:* The knowledge becomes such a part of you that you can use it automatically. You know it, you do it, and you teach it to others.

Upon reading this book, you may experience an awakening, as I did, to some truths and understandings you would never before have thought believable. If you are teachable, you may find yourself stepping through these four stages and, I hope, begin to awaken others to the powerful Self-Health truths you have embraced. I believe that if you are reading this book you are in all likelihood a teachable person who wants to improve your life and the lives of others. If so, step ahead with your skeptic's hat firmly on, but read with an open, teachable mind. The journey to Self-Health lies in the pages ahead.

*All truth passes through three stages.
First, it is ridiculed. Second, it is violently opposed.
Third, it is accepted as being self-evident.*

—ARTHUR SCHOPENHAUER,
GERMAN PHILOSOPHER

I **Thought** I Was **Dying**

He woke up from the dream of life
—Epitaph on a tombstone

It was my fortieth birthday. I took a good, hard look at myself. It was not a pretty sight. I thought of my dad. My father had been a great, Godly, hardworking man who had been strong and energetic most of his life. He was an incredible athlete in his thirties. I thought he was invincible. That is, until he became sick. He died at the age of fifty-seven, tired, overweight, broken by chronic illness and prescribed drugs that did more harm than good. I had vowed as I stood above his grave that I would not fall into the same fate. Yet as I looked in the mirror that day, I saw much of my father's disease in me, and, as you can imagine, it scared me to death.

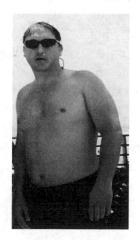

Fat and Fatter

I was only forty and felt like an old man. I was overweight and without energy. Fat, actually. You might say I was twice the man I wanted to be. I was able to make it through a day only by sheer grit and willpower. I felt so ill that I thought I was dying. Plagued with indigestion, I had morphed into a slob, into the out-of-shape, looking-older-than-I-actually-was, worn-out, beer-bellied type of person I had looked down on in my previous energetic, slim, and in-shape life. I thought of my future. I could easily see myself becoming a statistic. Was chronic illness, cancer, or a heart attack on the near horizon? And what of my family, whom I loved so dearly? Would they have to say goodbye to me far too early, just as I had when my own father died?

As I contemplated this man in the mirror (whose reflection seemed to barely fit in the mirror), I realized that unless something changed, I would have a larger waist next year, even less energy, and likely more health problems. I used to wear out clothes; now I grew out of them at a rate I could hardly believe. How could this have happened?

It happened one bite at a time. As the Irish scholar and educator Thomas Moffett said, "We are digging our graves with our teeth."

I have fond childhood memories of staying with my grandparents, helping them work in their organic garden, feasting with them day in and day out on the fresh vegetables and fruit they grew, the eggs they gathered, and the meat from the animals they raised. They had the best-tasting food I had ever experienced. They considered their food standard fare, but their eating and farming habits represented a way of life that would soon be crowded out and forgotten.

The Birth of Fake Food

In 1972, only eight years old, I was blissfully unaware that something devious was happening that would forever change the nature of food for me, my family, and every family in America. The FDA agreed to allow big food companies to advertise and sell "foods" that, for all practical purposes, were not really food at all. Imitation food, if you will, food-like substances, or as I like to call it, "fake food." According to Michael Pollan, the author of *The Omnivore's Dilemma*, in the 1800s states ruled that fake food, such as imitation butter, had to be dyed pink so no one would be fooled by it. But beginning in 1972 they could feed us this fake food and call it "bread, butter, milk or cheese," even if it wasn't really anything like what we had come to know as bread, butter, milk, or cheese.

Why would the FDA approve this, and why would large food companies want to do this? There are three reasons: (1) fake food is cheaper to make; (2) it lasts much longer on the shelf; and (3) its formulas, patents, and trademarks can be owned by one company, unlike real food. (Try to patent a peach!)

Remember Wonder Bread? It's so light, soft, and fluffy; it's even "enriched." ("Enriched" means they try to put back nutrients that processing has destroyed.) Wonder Bread, like so many modern breads, barely resembles the recipes Great-grandmom would have known. Compare the difference:

> ### Great-grandmother's Bread Ingredients
> *Stone ground whole wheat flour, yeast, water, honey, sea salt, olive oil*
>
> ### Wonder Bread (Processed Bread) Ingredients
> *Enriched white flour, water, wheat gluten, high fructose corn syrup, contains 2% or less of: soybean oil, salt, molasses, yeast, mono and diglycerides, ethoxylated mono and diglycerides, dough conditioners (sodium stearoyl lactylate, calcium iodate, calcium dioxide), datem, calcium sulfate, vinegar, yeast nutrient (ammonium sulfate), extracts of malted barley and corn, dicalcium phosphate, diammonium phosphate, calcium propionate (to retain freshness).*

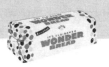

After reading the ingredients, you may "wonder" if it's bread at all. You should. In fact, a good rule of thumb is: **If you can't pronounce the names of the ingredients, don't eat it.**

A few years ago, a British judge in a tax case ruled that Pringles could not call themselves potato chips (or, in British parlance, potato "crisps") because only 42 percent of the chip is made of potatoes. The rest is made out of rice, flour, and other fillers.

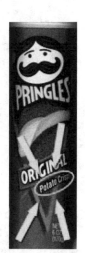

Ironically, Procter & Gamble (Pringles' makers) had actually argued in court that Pringles were *not* actually a potato chip so they wouldn't be subject to a 17.5 percent VAT tax. Initially, Pringles convinced the court they were not chips, but that ruling has now been overturned and Britain collects the tax revenue.

Yes, new and exciting fake foods have been produced, advertised, and dumped on the public, who have been buying these imitation foods in massive numbers. Doritos, Cheese Puffs, Twinkies, Pop-Tarts, Lucky Charms, and many other brands became popular new "foods" and could be found in almost every family's home and in most children's bellies. Television commercials featured product cartoon celebrities that became as well-known to the public as Walt Disney characters (Cap'n Crunch, Tony the Tiger, Ronald McDonald). Fast-food chains became a mark of civilization and popped up everywhere. We rapidly became what

Eric Schlosser aptly called "a fast food nation." America's diet changed so much that it became easier to find Big Macs and Cokes than to find an apple.

Faster Food Nation

Other changes soon followed. Mothers stopped wearing aprons and cooking meals. Eating out in restaurants, picking up take-out, or having fast foods delivered to the home became the rule, while eating home-prepared foods in family units became the exception. Fresh produce from the farm became a thing of the past, and most folks became too busy to even stop at the occasional farmers market that they passed along the road. Processed, frozen, instant, microwave, and packaged foods replaced fresh fruits and vegetables at my home and even at school. (I'm not kidding. I once asked a cafeteria worker where the vegetables were, and she pointed to the ketchup.) Convinced by junk food profiteers, schools everywhere put in snack and soda machines where profits from sales could be used as fundraisers. It seemed like kids' appetite for these fast foods was insatiable.

The Birth of the Big Mac

I too proudly joined the fast-food nation craze. My first job as a teenager

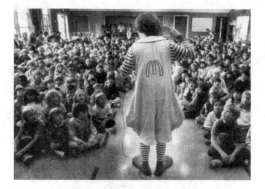

was at a McDonald's, and I eagerly sampled everything the creative geniuses from the fast-food giant's science labs could come up with to make fake food taste real. I witnessed the birth of the Big Mac, the Quarter Pounder with Cheese, the McChicken sandwich, and the now infamous Chicken McNuggets (the ultimate fake food). I was hooked. I had adopted a new lifestyle and eating habits that would follow me into adulthood. And I was not alone—millions of Americans were being seduced and led down the same path. We would march (or waddle) together into an unhealthy future.

The Fattening of America

In 1980, if you happened to be at a football game and stood at the top of the bleachers and gazed down at the crowd, you would have seen a few out-of-shape, overweight folks in the stands. Go to any football game today, a fast-food restaurant, a grocery store, or any public place, for that matter, and you will see that the majority of people are overweight and out of shape. There is simply no denying that America is getting fatter. It seems like there are fewer and fewer slim and fit people. In fact, the average adult today is 25 pounds heavier than in 1960, and the average child is 15 pounds heavier.

Yet while Americans are getting fatter, weight-loss clinics and businesses are booming. There are a few success stories, but think about it: these fat farms make money only if there are fat people. Their programs are usually hard to follow, they are almost always expensive, and they don't work for most people.

Fitness or Wellness?

You may be fit, but are you well? You may exercise regularly, run often, have big guns, tight glutes, and a six-pack to die for, and still be only one workout away from a heart attack or a cancer diagnosis. Remember Jim Fixx? He was the author of *The Complete Book of Running* and is considered by many to be the father of the modern fitness movement in America. He dropped dead at age fifty-two of a massive heart attack while running. Everyone was shocked. They were even more shocked when his autopsy revealed that fatty depos-

its had blocked 95 percent of one coronary artery, a second 85 percent, and a third 50 percent. He was fit, but not very well at all.

The body needs exercise, but exercise can't make us healthy. Exercise can only help a body that isn't overburdened with malnutrition from eating dead foods and toxins. If you are working out and exercising, you may look good, have energy, feel strong and upbeat, yet your body may be working overtime to handle the unhealthy effects of what you are eating.

Wellness is about feeding your cells and building your muscles with the most nutrient-dense foods on the planet. Your cells may look good, but what are they made of? How deep does your fitness go? For many, it's only skin deep. **You may look good but not be well. Fitness is a luxury, but wellness is a necessity.**

Seizing Self-Health

As I stared at the mirror on my fortieth birthday, contemplating my premature aging and imminent death by diet, I made a decision and said out loud, "I will not live another day like this!"

I determined to find a way to lose the weight, restore my energy, reclaim my body, and truly live my life as I was meant to live it: healthy and happy. I resolved that I would *not* fall prey to chronic illness as my father and millions of others had. I would not wake up one morning to find out that I had been diagnosed with cancer, heart disease, or diabetes. I would seize the day—this day. I would take control of my own health and destiny. From that moment everything in my life changed, and I began what I would soon call my Self-Health Revolution.

CHAPTER TWO

Sicker Than Our Parents

Without our health, there is no point . . . to anything.
Everett Mamor, French author and social commentator

Imagine a massive tsunami thousands of feet tall, barreling toward the United States at breakneck speed. In fact, the early waves have already begun to crest along our shores.

This approaching tsunami is the gigantic wave of Diabesity (obesity + diabetes).

For the first time in U.S. history, 35 percent of Americans are obese and diabetic. Even more frightening, this represents nearly a 25 percent increase in only three years (2008 to 2010). At this rate, somewhere between 50 and 70 percent of Americans will be obese in the next five to fifteen years. There is not a health care system in the world that will be able to handle this magnitude of sickness and subsequent medical costs. If this Diabesity tsunami remains unimpeded, it will likely destroy our health care system and potentially take down our fragile economy along with it.

It is mind-numbing to think that our generation is the first in American history to be sicker than the previous one. According to an article in the January 2010 *Journal of Pediatric Nursing*, this generation of children may be the first to have a life expectancy as much as ten years shorter than that of their

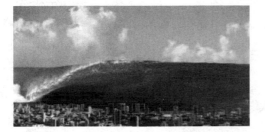

parents. By any measurement, America's health is failing. We spend more on health care than any society in the world, yet two-thirds of Americans are overweight (up 74 percent since 1991), over 20 million have diabetes (up 61 percent since 1991), and over 40 million have pre-diabetes (yet to be diagnosed). We still fall prey to heart disease at the same numbers we did thirty years ago, and the war on cancer, launched in the 1970s, has been a miserable failure. We are truly sicker than our parents, and certainly our grandparents.

Think about it. How many people do you know with diabetes or cancer or a heart problem or who are on prescribed medications? When I was growing up, these were the diseases of the elderly and the unfortunate few; now it's our mothers, fathers, sons, and daughters and, yes, even us.

Everybody's Getting One

One out of two men in this country will be diagnosed with cancer, and more than one out of three women. Picture this: in a room full of people, half of the men and at least a third of the women will develop some form of cancer—it's a fact. That's incredible, isn't it? We live in a modern medical world with perhaps the greatest intellectual civilization known to man, and yet in America 38 percent of us will die from cancer and 42 percent of us will be killed by a heart attack, heart disease, diabetes, or stroke. We know now that most of these diseases can be prevented, not by modern medicine but by specific choices we make as individuals. Yes, the power of prevention lies in the choices we make.

Not only are we sick, but we're tired. Fatigue is a problem for millions of Americans—30 million, to be exact. We wake up tired, we fall asleep watching a movie, we're too tired for sex, we doze off at the wheel or on the job. We try to combat fatigue with over-the-counter pills, energy drinks, high-priced Starbucks coffees, sugar, and even cocaine.

Feeling Our Pain

According to a 2011 Gallup poll, there's an even greater affliction, "the Hidden Epidemic," thus named because it was only recently known exactly how many people were suffering from it. What the researchers discovered was startling. The study revealed that 90 percent of Americans suffer from some specific pain on a regular basis (at least once a month), and 42 percent (90 million people) suffer from pain daily. If you are tempted to think this may be an exaggeration, just take a look at the pain medicine aisle in your local drug store. There's Tylenol, Advil, Motrin, Aleve, Anacin, Excedrin, Bayer, Bufferin, Ecotrin, Ascriptin, Capzasin, Doan's, Goody's, and BC Powders—just to name a few—with new ones appearing daily on a drug store shelf near you. Someone is making lots of money on our pain. What's your favorite pain reliever?

The Growing Dis-ease of Our Children

It is even more sad and discouraging to think about what is happening to our kids. If we are sicker than our parents, our children are surely becoming even sicker. The number of overweight children has virtually tripled in the past twenty years alone. Those of you perhaps a little older can easily confirm this by simply digging up and dusting off your old high school yearbook. Look at your classmates and compare them with kids in school now. You can see our kids getting fatter.

Because our children are fatter, a child born in 2000 has a 30 percent chance of developing diabetes, and we now know that 80 percent of diabetics will suffer from heart disease. In fact, autopsies of children as young as five revealed fatty deposits already building in their arteries, the beginning stages of heart disease. Wow!

Overall, almost 18 percent of children and adolescents have some sort of chronic health condition, nearly half of whom could actually be considered disabled to some degree. What is the grim prognosis for the next generation of Americans? Research reveals that an obese child is 70 percent more likely to become an obese adult. They are going to be fatter, have more chronic illnesses, be more asthmatic, have more cancer and more heart disease, and suffer from far more neurological disorders than any previous generation of Americans.

Why is this happening to our children? What can be done to protect the most innocent and vulnerable of us all? Does the answer lie within our grasp?

Tip of the Iceberg

Our nation is in real trouble, but the most troubling condition of all may be what we do not see. Like an iceberg, the greatest threat to our Self-Health is not what we can see but what lies beneath the surface. The tip of the iceberg is dramatically smaller than what is unseen just below the waterline. Just ask the captain of the *Titanic*.

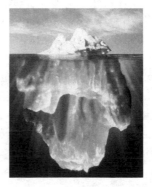

What if I told you that millions of Americans already have cancer and heart disease, and have for years, totally unaware of the growing danger out of sight, below the surface? They go to the doctor feeling fine and seemingly in good health, only to find out that their arteries are 80 percent clogged or stage 3 cancer is growing inside them.

We all know people who one day looked fine and the next day found out they were dying. Most people don't even know or understand what heart disease or cancer actually is, where it comes from, or how it works. I guess some don't want to know, but the truth is, most will become very familiar with it sooner or later.

Cancer Is You

Simply put, cancer develops when your body's normal cells freak out and go crazy. This cell insanity happens when cells do not get the right foods (nutrition) or are exposed to the wrong foods or toxins. In a healthy body, either such cells will die off or the body will step in and destroy them. Cancer cells not only do not die off; they duplicate and destroy the normal cells around them. Your body does not always recognize these cancerous cells as the enemy, so they keep growing until they consume everything and you die.

Cancer develops in three stages: ini-

tiation, promotion, and progression. You may have cancer for ten to twenty years without even knowing it. On average, it takes one year for a single cell to become twelve, six more years to become the size of a pencil point, ten or more years to even become detectable: the size of a pea. Millions have cancer right now but are years away from detection. And for the thousands who die of cancer every year, detection by modern medicine comes far too late. In fact, autopsies performed on people in their thirties and forties revealed tiny cancers growing in virtually every cadaver. It's not a question of whether we have cancer, but of which stage of cancer we are currently in.

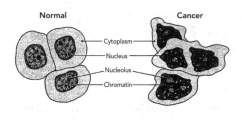

The Ultimate Clog

Heart disease, the other major killer, is even simpler to understand. Heart disease is basically the accumulation of bad foods (fats) on the inside of our arteries, the vessels that carry the blood through the body to the heart and brain. When we eat the wrong kinds of fat, they build up, much like the sludge in the drainpipe of your

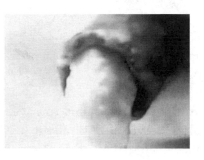

flow even while 80 percent blocked with sludge from fat. Many people have major blockage and are unaware of the invisible and life-threatening iceberg under their skin. A clogged artery is a ticking time bomb.

How Will You Die?

bathtub. The fat gradually sticks to the walls of your heart and arteries over time, causing blockages and clots that restrict and will eventually stop the flow of blood to your heart and brain. This condition can kill you quickly (by heart attack or stroke) or over a period of time (by heart and artery disease). About 25 percent of individuals who have heart attacks die the first time. Most were not even aware they had a heart condition. Many are familiar with the untimely death of the award-winning reporter Tim Russert of NBC News, who died a few years ago from his first known heart attack, although he had handily passed a heart exam and stress test just one month prior to the fatal attack.

Arteries are amazingly flexible creations. They can actually support blood

Let's face it: we are all going to die. Critics may disagree with many points made in this book, but on this point I am infallible. The human mortality rate is 100 percent. I don't have a crystal ball, but I can pretty much tell you right now how you are going to die. You cannot stop the Grim Reaper from coming, but what if I told you that you could probably control how and when he came? It's this simple: the World Health Organization shows that 90 percent of us will likely die in one of these four ways: cancer, heart attack, diabetes, or stroke.

What if I could show you a proven way to defend yourself and ward off these four killers? If I could show you a verified way to avoid cancer, heart disease, diabetes, stroke, and chronic illness, wouldn't you want that infor-

The Major Killers of Americans	Percent of Deaths
Heart attacks, diabetes, strokes	52%
All cancers	38%

If you're not sick, it doesn't mean you're healthy.

mation? How incredibly valuable would it be to you and to those you love the most?

There are basically two types of treatment people receive today: before-the-fact treatment and after-the-fact treatment. Many people wait until they get sick and then go to the doctor for after-the-fact treatment to save their health. Self-Health is about treating yourself before the fact, so that sickness never happens. After-the-fact treatment doesn't always work, and as you will see in the next chapter, the treatment may do more harm than good. Let me show you what I am talking about.

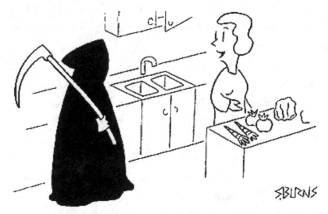

"Oh, how nice! You're just in time to cut the vegetables."

CHAPTER THREE

Myths of Modern Medicine

Whenever a doctor cannot do good,
he must be kept from doing harm.
—Hippocrates, father of medicine, 370 BC

Years ago, people said, "If you're healthy, you'll spend more money on your automobile mechanic than on your doctor." It used to be that way—back in 1975. To say medical care has become expensive is a dramatic understatement. The price of prescription medicine, doctor visits, hospital stays, and tests is increasing at a rate far beyond the price of gasoline. At least I know gasoline is good for my car. I am slightly more skeptical as to whether many modern medical practices have been good for our bodies.

Many of us are unintentionally on a plan to eat, drink, or swallow whatever food comes across our plate. Then we hope that the host of medical professionals will come to our res-cue if we become ill as a result of our eating lifestyle. Others are not quite convinced that there is actually a connection between what we eat, how we feel, and many diseases. Unlike with our car, for some unexplainable reason we are not quite sure if better food (fuel) really leads to better mileage and performance. But like gravity, it's there whether you believe it or not.

Good People in a Bad System

The truth is, medical professionals still do not understand what causes most diseases, nor do they know how to cure them. Physicians are primarily trained to treat symptoms, not to address causes, and certainly not to cure. They simply are not trained in nutrition and prevention. According to the sources I've consulted, out of 127 medical schools in the nation, 70 percent do not require courses on nutrition or prevention, and 30 percent do not even offer such courses. Doctors primarily know how to diagnose illness and prescribe medication, and, boy, do they know how to do that!

Has it ever annoyed you that, if you are late to the doctor's office, you get bumped from your appointment time or maybe even charged for your tardiness? And then, when you finally do manage to get back to what I call "the waiting waiting room" (the real waiting room), you have to wait for another thirty minutes. What's up with that? Well, don't blame your doctor just yet. It's not really his fault. Most doctors in our modern medical system are simply way too busy. Gone forever are the days (if we can remember them) of Marcus Welby, MD, when your doctor knew your name, your history, and your true health and had the time to focus solely on you. Many doctors are frustrated and even embarrassed by the modern medical system, but there is little they can do about it.

The Thirty-Second Diagnosis

It's actually worse than we thought. Get this: according to the *Journal of the American Medical Association,* the average interaction time between doctor and patient before interruption is a whopping twenty-three seconds. The same study revealed that the average doctor makes a diagnosis within the first thirty seconds of seeing a patient. Thirty seconds!

Doctors can spend as much time with you as they want, but they will not get paid by the insurance companies until they make a diagnosis. So in this "cattle call," insurance-driven system we have today, it's *Get them in, get them diagnosed, write a prescription, and get them out the door (and don't forget to take their money).*

One Drug Salesperson for Every Doctor

Have you noticed that the solution to your diagnosis is always a prescription drug? Doctors are trained in the art of writing prescriptions. Think about it: a doctor would be naked without a prescription pad. Have you ever seen a doctor without one?

There is no one who loves prescription-writing physicians more than the pharmaceutical companies. In fact, they have over 100,000 salesmen for every 120,000 doctors, tirelessly pursuing and enticing each physician to prescribe more and more of their wonderful drugs. They provide doctors with complimentary gourmet lunches, dinners, golf outings, trips, giveaways,

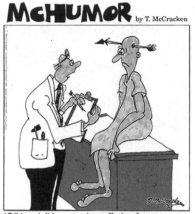

McHUMOR by T. McCracken

"Off hand, I'd say you're suffering from an arrow through your head, but just to play it safe, I'm ordering a bunch of tests."

and other freebies to the tune of $50 billion a year. (I guess I could get fired up to write a few prescriptions too.) Perhaps you have received a pen, a notepad, or some other trinket from one of these wonderful, caring, giving drug companies. It's just the way business gets done in our modern-day medical system.

All the while, there are no enticements or incentives for doctors to provide or promote nutrition, prevention, or wellness despite the evidence that proper nutrition and preventive tactics are the only way to avoid and even cure many diseases. There is simply no money to be made promoting nutrition and prevention. As they say, "It don't pay the bills."

Killing Sacred Cows

Some of my professors in graduate school would point out that as we learn new things, some of our sacred cows must die. A sacred cow is a person, custom, belief, or institution regarded as beyond criticism. The phrase *sacred cow* comes from India and the Hindu belief that cows are sacred. Interestingly, these sacred cows roaming the streets in New Delhi are now becoming sick and even dying because they are eating discarded plastic bags, one of the environmental scourges of Western civilization. (That's another book.)

The present health system has been built on its own mythology, a mythology that continues to feed and support that system. Here are the common myths and sacred cows of modern medicine:

1. Doctors always know what's best for the patient. (In fact, at times doctors don't even know or understand the problem!)
2. The doctor's diagnosis is the final word. (Be wary when doctor, nurse, and patient stop thinking and accept the prescribed remedy, which is usually dictated by the drug companies.)

3. Drugs and modern medical treatment can cure all diseases and medical conditions. (Many times the "cure" is worse than the illness, and often there are dangerous side effects.)

4. Modern medical tests will reveal the problem in time. (Many tests are unreliable and do not reveal disease before it's too late.)

The point is, if you are relying on modern medicine to save you from disease and premature death, you may be sorely disappointed. As you will see in the next chapter, this dependence on doctors and their drugs for our own Self-Health can be dangerous.

The doctor of the future will give no medicine but will interest his patients in the cause and prevention of disease.
—THOMAS EDISON

CHAPTER FOUR

The **Drugging** of **America**

(GETTING RICH FROM THE SICK)

We put drugs of which we know little, into bodies, of which we know less, to cure diseases of which we know nothing at all.
—Voltaire

What is the most profitable business in American history? The oil and gas industry? The computer industry? Technology (think Bill Gates and Steve Jobs)? How about real estate, the business in which Donald Trump made his billions? What about Wall Street and tycoons like Warren Buffett?

The answer is the pharmaceutical industry. Their profits dwarf those of many industries combined. In fact, the big oil companies, now hauling in record profits, regularly use the pharmaceutical companies' income to justify their own outrageous profits. In recent congressional hearings, an oil company executive countered accusations of greed in his industry by saying, "We are only making half the profit that the drug companies are making." So why is Congress investigating the oil companies and investment banks but not the drug companies? Read on and you'll have a good idea.

Wolves Among Sheep

In 1997 Congress passed a law that would forever impact the Self-Health of a country and soon the world itself. After the drug companies spent hundreds of millions of dollars in lobbying efforts (more than at any other time to that point in history), Congress decided it would be a good idea to allow them to advertise directly to the American people. Talk about letting wolves into the sheep's pen! Now the pharmaceutical salesmen could enter our homes through TV, radio, newspapers and magazines, and the Internet—following us everywhere. And what do you think was the result of this campaign to the American public?

Twenty years later doctors are writing 3.4 billion prescriptions a year. That's more than twelve prescriptions for every man, woman, and child in America. (And I'm not taking any, so someone has twenty-four prescriptions.) This is double the number from just ten years ago. Drug companies now spend over $18 billion a year in advertising and marketing, more than any other industry and more than any other period in history; in fact, one-third of all media advertising is paid for by drug companies. Don't believe me? Just turn on your favorite TV show and wait a few minutes, and you will see exactly what I am talking about. Their pitch will sound something like this:

> Are you tired? Are you sleepy? Trouble sleeping? Do you lie awake at night? Do you worry? Are you anxious? Do you have gas? Suffering from diarrhea? Constipated? Frequent urination? Going problem? Erectile dysfunction? Headaches? Arthritis? Restless leg? [What is that?] Do you get hungry? Do you eat too much? Do you get thirsty? Do you drink water? Do you breathe oxygen? Are you alive? Then we have a drug for you!

The Art of Self-Prescribing

There is no escape from this barrage. The pharmaceutical companies want all of us on some kind of drug for any reason they can possibly invent, and they are not very far from achieving just that. The commercials say, "Could _____ be right for you? Ask your doctor! Talk to your doctor! Call your doctor!" They call this self-prescribing. No longer do they need doctors to tell you what drug you should be taking. Why wait for the doctor when you can get the public to prescribe drugs for themselves? These smoothly crafted, almost seductive commercials do a much better job. And they are beautiful and beguiling, aren't they?

Sometimes I get the feeling the aspirin companies are sponsoring my headaches.

—V. L. ALLINEARE

CounterThink
"DISEASE MONGERS, INC."

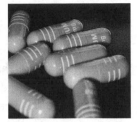

Picture a handsome young man and a virtual supermodel running hand-in-hand through a fresh field of the greenest grass you have ever seen. The grass is covered with a gorgeous array of flowers swaying in the breeze, butterflies bounce in the azure-blue sky, birds chirp happily as a comforting voice expounds on how wonderful your life will be once you have swallowed a Little Purple Pill. Amazing, isn't it?

What's even more amazing is the grace with which the commercials list, in a much softer voice and faster, the very bad things that might happen to you after you take the wonderful Little Purple Pill. These commercials are repeated thousands of times nationally and internationally.

Meet the Little Purple Pill

One night you are in your living room watching the news, when a serious-looking man on a cliff interrupts your evening to tell you, "I'm every man," and on an opposite cliff, separated from him by a chasm, a woman tells you, "I'm every woman," and together they proclaim, "We are every man and woman who has ever suffered from frequent persistent heartburn." Thundering waves crash, sunlight pierces cloud-filled skies, the chasm is filled, the once separate cliffs are connected, people from every race emerge to embrace and proclaim the good news of the capsule's coming. In awe, they look to the sky as millions of Little Purple Pills fall from the heavens. (I'm not making this up.) This sounds more like a description of the Second Coming of Christ than a drug commercial. What a gimmick!

For the drug companies it *has* been something of a Second Coming, if sheer profit means anything. The Little Purple Pill brings in a whopping $6 billion in revenue a year (as reported in 2004), more than any other prescription drug. At $4 a day, the Little Purple Pill has become so addictive for patients that doctors have jokingly dubbed it "purple crack."

What does this amazing "purple crack" really do? It shuts down acid-producing pumps used for digestion in the stomach (that's all), so that patients can resume eating fatty and spicy foods without experiencing pain, acid reflux, or GERD (gastroesophageal reflux disease). Who cares what's causing GERD? Just take the Little Purple Pill and forget about it. What's more important is that you can continue to eat all the chili you want without having to pay for it in physical discomfort. The drug companies have even arranged for the Little Purple Pill to be approved by the FDA for kids ages one to eleven. You should see what these children are now eating with the help of their Little Purple Friend.

The Small Print

If you or someone you love is taking or considering taking the Little Purple Pill, you might want to read the list of what they call "adverse drug effects" before popping some "purple crack." Here is a list (from their own website) of a few of the unfortunate side effects the pill can cause. Just so you know, in this list of bad side effects, I inserted all the easy-to-understand words in brackets.

Enlarged abdomen, back pain, chest pain, face swelling, fatigue, flu-like disorder, general swelling, leg swelling, malaise [feeling sick], pain, rigors [shaking], flushing [red skin], hypertension [high blood pressure], tachycardia [rapid heartbeat], goiter [swelling of the neck], bowel irregularity, constipation, esophageal disorder, frequent stools, gastroenteritis [stomach flu], dyspepsia [stomach pain], dysphagia [difficult swallowing], dysplasia [abnormal cell growth], epigastric pain, eructation [gas], hiccups, melena [black feces], mouth disorder, pharynx disorder, rectal disorder, tongue disorder, tongue edema [swelling], ulcerative stomatitis [gangrene ulcers of stomach], vomiting, earache, tinnitus [ear ringing], anemia [low red blood cells], hypochromic, cervical lymphadenopathy [lymph node swelling], epistaxis [nosebleed], leukocytosis, leukopenia, thrombocytopenia, bilirubinemia [bile in blood], abnormal hepatic function, glycosuria, hyperuricemia [acid in the blood], hyponatremia, thirst, weight increase, weight decrease, arthralgia [joint pain], arthritis, arthropathy, cramps, fibromyalgia [chronic pain], hernia, polymyalgia [muscle pain], rheumatica, anorexia, apathy, confusion, depression, dizziness, hypertonia [stiffness], nervousness, hypoesthesia [numbness], impotence [sexual dysfunction], insomnia [sleeplessness], migraines [headaches], paresthesia [pricking sensation], sleep disorder, somnolence [falling asleep], tremor [uncontrollable shaking], vertigo [dizziness], visual field defect, dysmenorrhea [painful menstruation], menstrual disorder, vaginitis, asthma, coughing, dyspnea [shortness of breath], larynx edema [swelling], pharyngitis, rhinitis [runny nose], sinusitis, acne, angioedema, dermatitis, pruritus, rash, erythematosus, inflammation, sweating, otitis media [middle ear inflammation], parosmia [smell loss], taste loss, taste perversion, abnormal urine, albuminuria, cystitis [bladder infection], dysuria [painful urination], fungal infection, hematuria [blood in urine], micturition frequency [frequent urination], moniliasis [yeast infection], genital moniliasis, polyuria, conjunctivitis, abnormal vision, duodenitis [inflammation of upper stomach], esophagitis [GERD], esophageal stricture, esophageal ulceration [ulcers], esophageal varices, gastric ulcers [stomach ulcers], gastritis [stomach inflammation], benign polyps or nodules [stomach tumors], Barrett's esophagus [long-term GERD damage], and mucosal discoloration.

This is a horrifying list! And did you notice that the very thing that the Little Purple Pill is supposed to cure, acid reflux (GERD), it can actually cause! They admit on their own legal documents that this marvelous Little Purple Pill can itself cause physical problems that you may never have had before popping their pill. Would you trade some acid reflux for, let's say, impotence or vaginitis? How about trading gas pain for some blood in your urine or loss of taste or smell? This is something they clearly don't want you to think about. But believe me, they wouldn't put this in print unless the risks were absolutely real and they were forced to share this information by law.

Can You Read Gibberish?

If the drug companies had their way, you would never see this list, much less read it. It's tucked away in a closet somewhere on their website. (I had to dig for it.) Even if you did see it, they're counting on your not being able to understand it. It's written almost entirely in medical gibberish, so when you do read it, you have no idea what it means. Remember, in the list of bad side effects you just read, I inserted all the easy-to-understand words in brackets. Wonder why the drug companies don't make it simpler for average people to understand?

Sometimes, in urgent situations, you might need to take a pharmaceutical drug, but you should always be careful to first read the small print and consult a medical dictionary.

Drugs, Marketing, and Mind Control

Now, I know some of you may be thinking, *Well, at least they do tell you in their TV ads that some bad things could happen to you if you take their drugs*. That's true, but most people have become so accustomed to hearing this list of very bad things that after a while, they hardly even notice what's being said anymore. It's called inoculation, and it's a mind-control technique. It's like the preventive shot the doctor gives to protect you, so that if the disease bug does comes around, you're not affected by it. In this case, when the list of very bad side effects is read, you have heard it so often that it no longer has any effect on you.

In fact, many people can no longer hear it at all. They only see the pretty pictures, the beautiful people, and the wonderful message of the Little Purple Pill. Although it is a form of hypnotism or mind manipulation, the pharmaceutical companies would prefer to call it effective advertising and marketing. Just think of how many of your friends and members of your own family have fallen under the spell of these ads. Perhaps you yourself have heeded the siren's call.

I guess they are right—just look how well the advertising blitzkrieg is working. Every day people by the hundreds of thousands, after watching their favorite drug commercial, run to their doctor's office to demand prescriptions for the Little Purple Pill. What's the doctor going to say? No? Of course not! He has been waiting for you for months. He is ready, armed to the hilt. He has $5 billion (all gifts from the drug companies) in brochures, pens, notebooks, paperweights, stress toys, and lots and lots of samples of the wonderful, perhaps magical Little Purple Pill. What a racket. Can this be legal?

Marketing Mother's Milk

Why did America jump on such a terrible treadmill of drugs, doctors, and devious advertising? How did all this get started? Unfortunately, like so many things I have been talking about, it's all about the money. Perhaps it began with something as simple as mother's milk.

Mother's milk is arguably the most healthful, nutrient-dense food on the planet. First of all, mother's milk is unique to each individual mother and each individual child. In essence, it is customized for the health of that particular little baby nursing on that particular breast. Every day the formula for that milk changes to meet the ever-evolving needs of an ever-evolving little baby. Amazingly complex, huh?

Mother's milk contains over a hundred ingredients that cannot be duplicated in the lab. It contains things like colostrum, which is loaded with nutrients and antibodies that protect the baby's body from disease. It seals the intestines, aids in digestion and absorption of nutrients, stimulates needed early bowel movements, and even relaxes the baby and helps it go to sleep. No one can dispute the nutritional superiority of mother's milk. Well, it did have one glaring weakness. You can't sell it! Unfortunately for the advertisers and marketers of big business, there is no money to be made on mother's milk. Or is there?

Better Than Mom's

In 1890 an enterprising capitalist named Henri Nestlé (yes, the guy who brought you chocolate milk, as well as ice cream, coffee, spices, pet food, and bottled water) thought it was time to get a piece of the mother's milk market. He created a replacement product: synthetic mother's milk, or mechanical milk, if you will.

The advertisements for this new mechanical milk made arrogant and audacious claims: "Best for Babies," the ads read. "Better for babies than mom's milk, for impure milk in hot weather is one of the chief causes of sickness among babies." They convinced not only mothers but many doctors as well through carefully crafted pamphlets and, of course, free mechanical milk samples. Real, natural, human mother's milk had met its match.

Health organizations around the world strongly encourage breastfeeding as the optimal source of nutrition for infants for the first year of life. Here's a short list: the World Health Organization (2002), the American Academy of Pediatrics (1997), the American Academy of Family Physicians (2003), the American Dietetic

Advertising may be best described as the science of arresting human intelligence long enough to get money from it.
—STEPHEN LEACOCK, CANADIAN ECONOMIST

Association (2001), the Institute of Medicine (1991), the Life Sciences Research Organization (1998), the U.S. Department of Health and Human Services (2000), Health Canada, and the Canadian Pediatric Society (1998).

Yet in spite of such support, the vast majority of infants in the United States are fed human milk substitutes. The power of advertising and marketing by greedy companies is not to be underestimated or ignored. If these companies can get mothers who dearly love their children to give up feeding them the most nutritious food in the world, what else can they do? The possibilities are endless.

A Whole New World for Eight-Year-Olds

How about cholesterol drugs for eight-year-olds? Unbelievably, CNN recently reported that the American Academy of Pediatrics issued a statement, with the approval of the FDA, strongly urging parents of overweight and obese

children as young as eight years old to immediately put their kids on a cholesterol drug to avoid future heart disease and heart attacks. Can you believe that? Have they ever thought of changing what our children are eating? I can already see the twinkle in the eyes of pharmaceutical executives in boardrooms across America as they fantasize about advertising these drugs to a whole new market, eight-year-old children (perhaps on Saturday morning cartoons).

No One Cares About the Cause

Imagine that one day you are walking barefoot in the yard and accidentally step on a very sharp nail. The nail pierces your skin, lodging deeply into your foot. Quickly you get in your car and race to the emergency room. Once you arrive, you hobble through the hospital doors, frantically scribble through the mandatory paperwork, and make your way to the infamous waiting room, where the doctor finally arrives

> *People think the FDA is protecting them. It isn't. What the FDA is doing and what people think it's doing are as different as night and day.*
> —HERBERT LAY,
> FORMER FDA COMMISSIONER

to look at your gruesome, self-inflicted wound. He carefully examines the now bloody nail that is deeply jammed into your swelling foot. "Hmmm," he says, "I think I have just the thing for you." He then reaches for his prescription pad and pen, and as he writes he says, "This codeine is really going to do the trick. It will dull the pain. You're going to feel so much better. You won't even notice the nail is there."

Upon hearing this, you feel a little confused and uncomfortable and say, "Hey, Doc, what about the nail?" The doctor calmly and confidently replies, "Let's not worry about the nail too much right now, okay? Let's focus on getting you feeling better. Then we might have a look into this 'nail business.'"

At that moment, mangled foot or not, if you don't think about running out of the waiting room or at least calling the nurse for a new doctor, having a nail shoved in your foot may be the least of your worries.

As absurd and sad as this story is, this scenario plays out in doctors' offices, hospitals, and medical centers all around the country. Millions of patients visit America's medical institutions every day. They come with all kinds of chronic illnesses and diseases, hoping for a cure, only to discover that the focus of our medical community is not on cures or causes and certainly not prevention. The feeling seems to be, *Let's just slap a drug on it and make the symptoms go away. Who really has the time to figure out what's causing it, much less curing it?* Of course, I am being sarcastic here. I know many doctors and health care professionals care about their patients, and I believe most are good people simply stuck in a bad system. Yet the sad truth is that millions of Americans walk out the door of our medical facilities every day, drugged up and destined to live decades of their lives with the proverbial nail still deeply lodged in their foot.

Who's Minding the Drug Store?

Is there anyone minding the drug store in America? How do all these drugs get on the market anyway? That would be the responsibility of the FDA, the U.S. Food and Drug Administration. This is the same group of folks who brought us imitation food (fake food) in the 1970s and drug advertisements in the 1980s (such as the Little Purple Pill). The FDA has long been suspected of having curiously cozy relationships with the folks it has been charged with regulating. Their management and oversight of the pharmaceutical industry is no exception. In fact, many former FDA commissioners have either worked for or now work for major drug companies. As much as 50 percent of the current funding for new drug approval processes is paid directly to

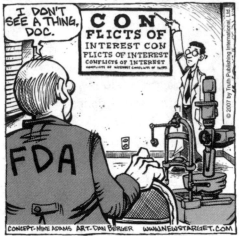

COUNTERTHINK "FDA VISION TEST"

jects. There are three phases of trials that the FDA puts a drug through in order to prove the drug is safe so it can be made available to the market. Look at the tiny number of people who are typically tested:

Phase 1: 20 to 80 people
Phase 2: 100s of people
Phase 3: 1,000 to 3,000 people

At best, several thousand people are tested before a drug is released to impact over 300 million mothers, fathers, sisters, brothers, grandparents, and children. Released to be shot over the airways and aimed at every home, every car, every computer, and every publication. Released to the most sophisticated and greedy Madison Avenue marketers ever known, profiteers who create ads so compelling that they drive thousands from their homes to waiting rooms where doctors are indeed waiting with open arms, gifts, and free samples. What can happen when you release a drug tested by so few and sent out with such vigor?

the FDA by the drug companies themselves, some $400 million annually. What's even more disturbing is how these new drugs are tested.

Who's Failing the Drug Test?

How many pregnant mothers, babies, middle-aged and elderly people are tested with a new drug before it's released to the public? Ten thousand? Five thousand? A thousand? Try none. The FDA and drug companies have no idea how their drugs will affect these groups of people. Only 22 percent of the people who are tested are women; most of those tested are young men. Sorry, ladies, this selection process means you may be in for an "adverse drug effect."

What's even more astounding is the relatively small number of test sub-

Death by Health Care

What can happen? Vioxx can happen. To millions of Americans who suffered daily from pain, Vioxx was a "miracle." Used by 20 million people, endorsed and promoted by the medical establishment and celebrities like the Olympic figure skating champion Dorothy Hamill, Vioxx became the most widely prescribed pain medication in the world. With annual sales of over $2.5 billion it was one of the best-selling drugs of all time. From the time the FDA approved it, Vioxx was hailed as a miracle drug that could reduce all kinds of pain without causing stomach problems experienced with older drugs such as aspirin, Advil, and Aleve. Merck, the drug company that owned Vioxx, was regarded as the industry's ultimate science-driven company, corporate America's greatest keepers of ethical standards, and was voted Best Company to Work For five years in a row.

Shoot the Messenger

Then, in 2004, Dr. David Graham, a lead researcher in the FDA's Office of Drug Safety, revealed that as many as 140,000 patients in the United States may have suffered serious heart damage from taking Vioxx, and that many of those cases may have been fatal. His team found more than 8,000 cases of coronary heart disease and just over 1,500 incidents of heart attack deaths. Amazingly, patients taking Vioxx had a 34 percent greater chance of coronary heart disease.

It gets worse. The study was originally slated to be published in November 2004; however, Graham says, the FDA threatened to dismiss him if the study appeared in a medical journal. Unbelievable, isn't it? Who's minding the drug store?

A memo from Edward Scolnick, the head of Merck's research and development, clearly showed that management knew in 2000 that Vioxx could cause serious heart problems, but they spent the next four years trying every way they could to not acknowledge it. They tried to intimidate researchers who wanted to study Vioxx's cardiovascular effects, telling the department chairman of a Stanford University researcher—who was giving lectures that Merck and others sponsored—that his career could "flame out" if his lectures raised questions about the safety of Vioxx. Merck trained their sales reps to play "dodge ball" with phy-

There's many a mistake made on purpose.
—THOMAS HALIBURTON,
CANADIAN AUTHOR

sicians who brought up any questions about Vioxx's harmful cardiovascular side effects.

Drugs, Money, and Murder

To date, not one person from Merck or the FDA has been punished or charged with any wrongdoing. Merck has had to pay about $1 billion in lawsuits, fines, and settlements but has not had to admit to any liability or wrongdoing. It appears Merck still pocketed billions from $12 billion in revenues it collected during Vioxx's life cycle. A stunning profit from selling a drug that cost thousands of lives and harmed millions, many of whom are still suffering to this day.

Vioxx should stand as a stark warning to all who would put their faith in the faulty U.S. medical system, the deceptive pharmaceutical industry, and the corrupted Food and Drug Administration. Yet as we speak, millions are mindlessly handing over the fate of their Self-Health to these same faulty institutions.

OOPS . . . That Wasn't Supposed to Happen

I have talked about heart attacks and cancer, but guess what the third leading cause of death in America is today? Strokes perhaps? Diabetes? (Hold on to your hats.) Unbelievably, the third leading cause of death in America is actually health care. That's right. Health care kills over 225,000 people every year. Medical errors, surgery screwups, hospital blunders, and hospital-borne infections are all on the list, but the number one death-by-health-care killer is by far prescription drugs. Over 106,000 people die every year from taking their prescriptions in normal doses, exactly as directed by their doctors. (This does not include thousands who accidentally took the wrong dosage.)

These deaths, one of the "adverse side effects," kill more people each year than breast cancer and colon cancer combined. Isn't it ironic that in America we have all of these foundations, nonprofits, fundraisers, and telethons

> ## A hospital is no place to be sick.
> —SAMUEL GOLDWYN,
> ACADEMY AWARD–WINNING PRODUCER

to raise money and awareness about breast cancer and colon cancer, and yet more people die each day from taking medication as prescribed by their doctors? Perhaps there is room for one more lifesaving cause in America. The slogan could be "Just say no to prescription drugs."

As you can see in the death-by-health-care chart, we cannot afford to rely on health care for our Self-Health. The reason pharmaceuticals kill more than 106,000 people each year is because these drugs are poisons. Any drug you will ever meet has a long list of very bad side effects for one simple reason: they are toxic and harmful to your body and should be taken only when there are no other options.

So be careful of what you are putting into your body, even if the FDA, the drug companies, and your doctor say it's good for you. They have been wrong before and probably will be again in the very near future.

Cause of Death	Deaths
Diseases of the Heart	710,000
Cancer	553,091
Medical Care	225,400
Stroke	167,661
Chronic Respiratory Disease	122,009
Accidents	97,900
Diabetes	69,301
Flu and Pneumonia	65,313
Alzheimer's Disease	49,558

Death By HealthCare	
Medication Errors	7,400
Unnecessary Surgery	12,000
Preventable Errors in Hospitals	20,000
Hospital Borne Infections	80,000
Adverse Drug Effects	106,000

Source: "Medical Errors: A Leading Cause of Death," The Journal of the Ameican Medical Association (JAMA) 284, no.4, July 26, 2000, written by Barbara Starfield, MD, MPH, of the Johns Hopkins School of Hygiene and Public Health.

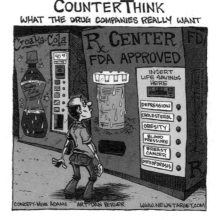

CHAPTER FIVE

If It Can Happen **to Me,**
It Can Happen **to You**

In order to be a realist, you must believe in miracles.
—David Ben Gurion, the first prime minister of Israel

Perhaps you woke up this morning with a small headache, your back was a little stiff, or your energy level was a bit lower than it was ten years ago. You were likely thinking, "I guess this is just what happens when you get old." People seem to think that as you get older you should feel bad and there's nothing you can do about it. I am here to say in no uncertain terms that it doesn't have to be this way. There is a difference between getting older and aging. Years go by, birthdays pass, but you don't have to age at the same rate. You can be physically younger than your actual age.

I know this is true. I know it because I have experienced it. Right now, at this moment, I am truly in the best shape of my life, and I owe it all to the teach-ings of Self-Health I am now shar-ing with you. Let me tell you how my Self-Health Revolution came about. If it happened to me, it could happen to you as well.

I was only forty years old, tired, over-weight, and on the verge of a chronic disease, perhaps a heart attack, or even worse, cancer. I had tried so many dif-ferent things to get healthy: the Atkins diet, Weight Watchers, South Beach, trainers, coaches, books, tapes—anything I could think of. I remember how hopeful I was when FedEx deliv-ered the box of food from Nutrisys-tem. I was so excited to open my first breakfast packet. I couldn't believe it: powdered eggs. (Talk about dead food.) These bad diet experiences only con-vinced me of my inevitable doom.

Then one especially painful day, I was thinking about the death of my beloved father, my hero. I recalled how quickly he went from athletic health to chronic illness and then death at the young age of fifty-seven. Here I was, speeding down the same road, knowing full well where it would end.

I decided in one powerful moment to get off this fatal path and take control of my own health. I determined that I would not stay fat, get sick, or die young. I suddenly realized the world doesn't care if I live or die. The FDA, with all of its regulations to protect me; the big food companies feeding me their fake foods; the pharmaceutical industry selling me syringes and purple pills; the doctors, hospitals, and medical centers pushing their diagnoses, prescriptions, and surgeries—none of them would or could come to my rescue and save my life. I could blame them or my genes, my culture or my schedule, my upbringing or so many other easily manufactured causes, but in that moment of clarity, I realized that dead men do not make excuses or apologies. I wanted to live. I wanted a full, healthy, vibrant life and not to waste a day that God had given me. What could I do with twenty more years, or even forty? That's a whole new life. There was so much more I wanted to do, see, share, and experience. My intense desire to live led me to the information in this book, this information fed my beliefs, and my new beliefs drove me to take action.

The Human Sponge

I began reading everything I could on Self-Health, the idea of taking control of your own health. I read over a hundred books, studied a thousand websites, listened to countless videos, CDs, and tapes. I made calls to experts all over the country, traveled hundreds of miles to talk with some of the smartest people I could find. They say, "When the student is ready, a teacher appears." I became a human sponge soaking up every bit of knowledge I could find on Self-Health.

To my dismay, what I initially found was confusing. Some experts contradicted other experts. There were so many diets, philosophies, gurus, products, elixirs, vitamins, drinks, books, tapes, commercials—it was unending. I was so confused and frustrated that I wanted to quit my quest and return to the comfort of my fat farm lifestyle. But then I decided that I would do something unique, original, and very uncommon these days. I decided to think for myself, to rely on my own common sense, and to put everything to the test for myself. Thus the idea of Self-Health was born.

I began to write down all of the ideas that made sense to me, things that appealed to my common sense.

> *Common sense is very uncommon.*
> —HORACE GREELEY

Then I started to try them, to put them into practice and see if they worked. The first thing I did was to cut back on eating red meat and later even chicken. I was used to eating about 80 percent meat and (maybe) on a good day 20 percent vegetables. (I never ate fruit.) Many times my only veggies were the tomatoes and lettuce found on a McDonald's Quarter Pounder with Cheese, which I would pick up at the drive-thru a few times a week or more. Once I discovered where my meat was really coming from, how poisoned and fatty it truly was (up to 500 percent more fat than grass-fed meat), I slowly stopped eating it.

Eventually I ate only organic, grass-fed, free-range beef and chicken and a lot of wild-caught fish, all of which I found at Whole Foods Market, local farmers markets, and other health-conscious grocery stores. It was more expensive, but cheaper than future hospital bills, chemotherapy, or funeral costs. I began to reintroduce myself to the fruits and vegetables I had known and loved as a child on my grandparents' organic farm. What a reunion that was!

I woke each morning and ate blueberries, raspberries, strawberries, cherries, grapefruit, kiwis, apricots, bananas, pineapple, and mangos. I had forgotten there were so many wonderful, juicy flavors. I created an incredible drink which I now call the Self-Health Smoothie, and I will soon pass this recipe along to you. I made salads that were out of this world, with lettuces,

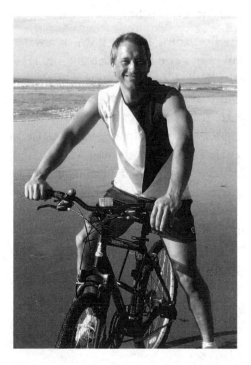

herbs, and vegetables that would fill my mouth with incredible new flavors and my body with outrageous nutrients. My salads are packed with so much healthful food that one serving will produce more nutrition than most people see in a week or even a month of eating.

My friends, my family, and everyone I knew were in shock at my improved health, the changes I had made in my lifestyle, and the weight I had lost. For the first time since my early youth, I began to feed my body living foods. Wow, did it ever change my life! This was the beginning of what I would soon call my Self-Health Revolution.

The Incredible Shrinking Belly

The first thing I noticed was my waist. My pants got looser and looser. Happily, I had to keep adjusting my belt, and eventually had to buy a new belt altogether. I went from a size 36 waist all the way down to a 31, the size I was when I was twenty-five. My bloated, fat, double-chinned face melted into the thin, recognizable neck and cheeks of my youth. I began to experience more energy, more excitement, more hope, more joy, and more peace about my future.

I no longer fell asleep during movies, at my desk staring at the computer, or while lying in bed waiting to make love. (Self-Health helps in that department too.) My bathroom experiences became pleasant, not painful. I didn't feel like reaching for Rolaids, Tums, or Pepto-Bismol after each meal. Aches and pains that had consistently greeted me each morning and throughout the day had disappeared. My hair, which had been thinning and falling out, started to grow so fast I had to get it cut every few weeks. Wrinkles and crow's feet that made me look so old and sometimes even elderly faded. I had the energy now to start walking, even running and working out. Flab disappeared, toned muscles emerged, the body of my youth was returning, and it felt unbelievable.

All of this started happening within months of starting my Self-Health Revolution. I now believed. Living foods do make a difference. How could I have been so foolish all those years to think that they wouldn't?

What had opened my eyes? What had finally made the difference for me? What happened to me was simply this: the pain of staying the same had become too great. Let me explain.

The Pain of Staying the Same

Change is frightening and can be painful. Many of us would rather die than change. That's why we sometimes see people eating Big Macs in their hospital room just hours after open-heart surgery. They would rather die than change, and probably will. We fear change because we are under the false impression that change will take away something we really need and love, something we have become deeply dependent upon for some bit of pleasure.

Have you heard the term *comfort food*? Millions of Americans turn to food not out of hunger but for comfort. We eat the foods that make us feel safe, warm, loved, full, and familiar. When we do this, we are living to eat, not eating to live. We hold on to these comforting, pleasing foods much like a child clutches a security blanket. We believe that these foods are good for us, or at least they are not nearly as bad as life would be without them. The truth is, if we were not so afraid of letting go, we might have a chance of experiencing something far superior.

Have you ever tried to hold on to something that you thought you really wanted and needed, but ended up losing it anyway? Then, later on, you were actually thankful that you lost it? That's happened to me so many times. In those cases, the security blanket was ripped away from me. At the time I had no choice in the matter, but now, in retrospect, I am glad that it was taken away. My point is this: sometimes you have to decide for yourself to put down the plate of comfort food in order to pick up the platter of living food. Once

you take the risk and really do it, you will wonder what took you so long.

I put down my old lifestyle of comfort foods when the burden of carrying around dead foods (in the form of fat, fatigue, and depression) became too painful. People change when the pain of staying the same outweighs the pain of changing.

Getting Off Our Nail

I am reminded of a story of a traveling, door-to-door salesman who, out of boredom and curiosity, decided to venture down an unpaved, gravel road. He could see a mailbox from where he was standing, and as he walked he came upon an old wooden shack, not much of a house. He stepped on the front porch and knocked on the door. After he knocked several times, a gentle, kind-looking old man came to the door. "Can I help you?" he asked. The salesman began the pitch he had delivered on thousands of front porches before. He was suddenly interrupted by what sounded like the painful yelping of an old hound dog. He asked the old man, "What the heck is that?" The old man replied, "That's just my hound dog, just ignore him. Go on with your pitch, son." A few more minutes passed. The dog erupted even more loudly, as if in more pain than before. The old man assured him that everything was okay and urged him to continue. This went on for a good fifteen minutes. Frustrated and worried, the young salesman looked intently at the old man and asked, "What in the Sam Hill is wrong with your dog, sir?" The old man calmly replied, "Oh, don't worry about him. That old hound dog is just sitting on a nail. When it gets to hurting too bad, he'll get up."

When it becomes too painful for us to keep doing what we are doing, we make changes. Sometimes you have to remind yourself just how painful life will be if you don't change.

So I started asking myself painful questions: What if I keep living this way? What if I keep eating this nasty food? How am I going to feel? What will I look like? What if I get even fatter? Do I like what I see when I look in the mirror? How do my kids view me? What if I become chronically ill? What if I get cancer? What if I drop dead of a heart attack? What's going to happen to my children, my wife, and my family? Will they suffer without me? What will I miss out on that I had hoped to experience?

Believe me, these questions were

painful, but they were necessary because they revealed a potential reality: If I didn't change, I would die. Maybe not in the coming weeks or months or even years, but I would die, much younger than I was intended to and perhaps without fulfilling my purpose, dreams, and goals.

So I forced myself to ask those hard questions. I ratcheted up the pain of staying the same by reading articles, books, whatever I could get my hands on, until one day the scales tipped and the pain of changing seemed a small price to pay to save my life. "Anything is better than this," I thought. So I dropped my dead comfort foods and eagerly picked up living foods. I know it sounds simple and immediate, but it wasn't. For most of us, change takes time, and it did for me as well.

Feed Your Beliefs and Starve Your Doubts

Even now, I find myself occasionally grabbing a greasy wing, a fried Tater Tot, or even a sugary donut, but as my belief grows in the power of living

---

You can't hire someone else to do your pushups for you.

—JIM ROHN,
BUSINESS PHILOSOPHER

You are the average of five people you spend the most time with.

—JIM ROHN,
BUSINESS PHILOSOPHER

foods and Self-Health, my desire for those things lessens. It is important to feed your belief. When you start making changes, even if they are changes for the good, many people around you will question your new choices and lifestyle. They don't understand why you are eating an apple rather than a hamburger or drinking water instead of a Coke. That's why it's important to surround yourself with positive thoughts, beliefs, and people. Read everything you can on Self-Health. Listen to CDs and tapes. Look for others who are trying to do the same thing you are. Carry this book in your car, purse, briefcase, or coat pocket, and read it throughout the day. Build your beliefs, and they will give you the power to take action, make changes, and sustain those new patterns over a long period of time.

Failure Isn't Fatal

You will, as they say, fall off the wagon. (At times, you may jump off.) It's important to give yourself permission to cheat from time to time. Let yourself taste some tempting dead foods,

or have a dead-foods day, because after you are hooked on living foods you will never go back for very long. Don't make everything off limits (smell it, touch it, taste it), or you will want it even more. No one is flawless when it comes to Self-Health, and that's okay and normal. Certainly don't be judgmental toward others who don't have your same Self-Health beliefs.

I mess up all the time on vacation, when I eat out with friends, when I get too busy at work, when I'm running to make an appointment. Sometimes it's difficult and challenging to get living foods. Don't worry or become discouraged if you mess up. Just get right back to it as soon as you can. If I have a bad day or week, I just come right back to Self-Health because I believe in it, my body now craves it, and I know it's the only thing that will save me. I can't help it now because it's part of who I am.

Don't focus on your mini-failures. Choose not to listen to self-defeating suggestions. Picture yourself winning, getting fit, looking younger, feeling great. Entertain only thoughts that confirm your success, and declare war

> *As a man thinks in his heart, so is he.*
>
> —KING SOLOMON

on everything else. Just think about how great those fruits and veggies are going to taste, how they'll make you look, and how you're going to feel, and hurry right back to your Self-Health lifestyle.

Roger Bannister and the Four-Minute Mile

On May 6, 1954, Roger Bannister did what was believed to be impossible. He became the first human ever to

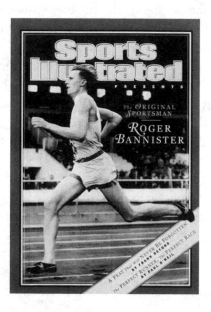

run a mile in less than four minutes. His time was 3 minutes 59.4 seconds. Before that windy British day, everyone thought a four-minute mile was scientifically and physically impossible, as no one had ever come close.

Although Bannister's feat was nothing short of a sports miracle, the breakthrough events that followed were even more amazing. Within fifty-six days, John Landy broke Bannister's record at 3 minutes and 57.9 seconds in Finland. Within a few short years over sixteen other runners had also accomplished the impossible, breaking the four-minute mile. Today the current world record is 3:43.13, set by Hicham El Guerrouj of Morocco on July 7, 1999, a full sixteen seconds faster than Bannister (a light-year in running).

What made a physical impossibility become a reality for so many people in such a short period of time? What changed? Did reality change? Did these humans suddenly become faster in only fifty-six days? The only thing that could have changed that quickly was their perception of reality. The four-minute mile was impossible because they believed that it was. When that belief was proved false, suddenly other great runners were able to do it. Today it is considered commonplace for a runner to break the "impossible" four-minute barrier.

Do You Have a Thinking Problem?

As you face the barriers to your own Self-Health, success may seem impossible. It may be hard to imagine yourself fit, thin, energetic, and healthy. You may doubt your own ability to put down dead foods and pick up these new living foods. Recognize, as Roger Bannister did, that your belief in Self-Health is more important than any one thing. Henry Ford once said, "Whether you think you can or think you can't, you're right." We must protect our thoughts at all costs. Our beliefs give us the power to keep going when nothing else can. Thoughts and beliefs have given birth to so many impossible ideas and accomplishments that now seem obvious or commonplace. Sometimes things have to be believed to be seen.

So vow to not allow limiting thoughts and beliefs to invade your Self-Health hopes and dreams. For free tools on how to starve your fears and feed your faith, see our website, www.SelfHealthRevolution.com now!

> *Impossible is a word to be found only in the dictionary of fools.*
> —NAPOLEON BONAPARTE

CHAPTER SIX

Diet Designed for Disease

We are digging our graves with our teeth.
—Thomas Moffett, Irish scholar and educator

Each time you sit down to have a meal you are making a life-and-death decision. With each meal, you are at a fork in the road. One fork leads to vibrant fitness, energy, disease-free health, and full life. The other fork leads to fatigue, weight problems, chronic illness, and perhaps even premature death. Sorry to be so blunt, but as they say, reality bites, especially if you are biting into the wrong food. Choose the fork with the right food at the end of it, and it will make all the difference.

Killing Us Slowly

In the sixteenth century something called "slow poisoning" became a popular phenomenon and even socially acceptable among certain groups of people. It is the practice of poisoning someone over a long period of time, so slowly that the poisoned individual seems to be simply dying of an unknown disease or illness. Most onlookers and victims never made the connection between the "slow poison" and the victim's poor health. Our generation is not all that different; our "slow poison" of choice today is the food we put in our mouths. Perhaps that's why Americans rank among the lowest of industrialized nations in terms of life expectancy.

Have you noticed what people eat today? It's amazing to me that we can manage to stay alive after eating some of the things that we eat. For example, recently I heard they were serving

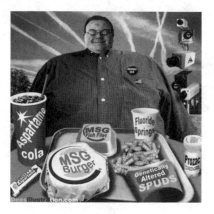

a new dessert at the state fair called "fried Coke." Yes, they actually pour Coke into a deep fryer full of grease, then put it into a cup and top it with whipped cream and sugar—and of course a cherry, because fruit is good for you. That might be an example of "fast poison." Fast or slow, we Americans are killing ourselves in three ways: breakfast, lunch, and dinner.

The Death of Food

As I said earlier, in 1973 the FDA, Congress, and the big food companies managed to get the imitation food laws tossed out, telling us that fake foods could be even better for us than the real thing. That was just the beginning of the fall of food. After convincing us to eat their fake foods, large food manufacturers continued to seek cheaper and cheaper ways to manufacture products and make even more money. They began taking traditional

whole foods and refining or processing them. As you know, the Wonder Bread (I wonder if it's bread?) of today is not our great-grandmother's bread. Big food manufacturers have taken the whole wheat kernel (where bread used to come from) and squeezed out up to 90 percent of the nutrients with giant rollers in order to create a product that is cheaper to produce and has a much longer shelf life. Who cares if it has little or no nutritional value, or if eating it actually does bad things to our body, as long as it makes the companies more money?

Think about all of the processed foods that litter our grocery store shelves today. Our great-grandparents would not recognize them: white bread, white sugar, white flour, white rice, white pasta, margarine, mayonnaise, frozen dinners, freeze-dried meals, cereals, skim milk, juices from concentrate, canned biscuits, canned Cokes, fried foods, prepackaged meals, Pop-

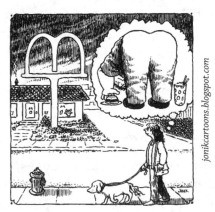

jomikcartoons.blogspot.com

Tarts, PAM, and, of course, Pringles and one thousand other processed foods we know all too well. Remember, a processed food is any food that has been altered from its natural state. Today that's most of the foods we eat. And in almost every case, these processed foods are not only robbed of nutrition (causing malnutrition), but they also carry harmful toxins—the two causes of most diseases.

Attack of the White Menace

The greatest culprits of the processed poisons are what Dr. Mark Hyman, in his book *UltraPrevention,* calls the White Menaces: white sugar, white bread, white fat, white pasta, and white rice. All of these white menaces contain sugar or convert immediately to sugar once in the body. The sugar that is not used is converted to fat. These white foods are bleached and stripped of all nutrients. They are found on grocery store shelves and in pantries across America. Our white food addiction has accelerated to a record-breaking roll.

Smothered and Covered in Syrup

Surveys conducted by the U.S. Department of Agriculture reveal that the average American is consuming twenty teaspoons of white sugar per day. Soft drinks today contain about nine teaspoons of sugar per twelve-ounce can

alone, and Americans drink seven times more soft drinks than we did just a few decades ago. New studies say soft drinks are the number one cause of America's obesity epidemic. The man-made form of sugar found in soda, high-fructose corn syrup (HFCS), contains more calories and "bad" fats than even natural sugar. HFCS has replaced regular sugar in most products today. Why? It's cheaper to manufacture. Look at almost any processed food label and you will see it listed, usually as the second or third highest ingredient. It is six times sweeter than sugar. It does not act the same way as regular sugar in the body. HFCS is processed more like fat in the body. Some experts believe that it actually converts to fat faster and more readily than regular sugar. It also may contribute to sugar cravings because of its supersweet flavor.

Things "Grow Better" with Coke (as Pesticide)

America's sweet tooth may explain why the nation's single biggest selling "food" is now soda. The Atlanta-based Coca-Cola Company sells over 1 billion bottles and cans of the stuff every day. Guess what the number two ingredient in Coke is? That's right! High-fructose corn syrup. But that's not all that's in it.

Just a few years ago one of the

United Nations' organizations and the Centre for Science and Environment found the presence of four extremely toxic pesticides and insecticides in Coke and Pepsi products in India: lindane, DDT, malathion, and chlorpyrifos at levels up to thirty-six times the acceptable amounts. This daunting discovery was revealed when Indian farmers were using The Real Thing to kill bugs on their crops. Instead of paying hefty fees to international chemical companies for patented pesticides, they were spraying their cotton and chili fields with Coca-Cola.

It turns out that things grow better with Coke, and it's a lot cheaper than buying pesticides from Monsanto, Shell, or Dow. So many farmers began using Coke as a pesticide that it became a powerful profit source for Coca-Cola bottlers in India. Gotu Laxmaiah, an Indian farmer, applied the beverage to several fields of cotton. He was delighted with his new cola spray. "I observed that the pests began to die after the soft drink was sprayed on my cotton," he told the *Deccan Herald*, an Indian newspaper.

A spokesman for Coca-Cola in Atlanta said, "We are aware of isolated cases where farmers may have used soft drinks as part of their crop management routine. Soft drinks do not act in a similar way as pesticides when applied to the ground or crops. There is no scientific basis for this and the use of soft drinks for this purpose would be totally ineffective." Totally ineffective? I guess that's why Indian farmers have paid out so much of their hard-earned cash to use Coke products as pesticides.

Although several Indian state governments stepped in and banned Coke, the bans on Coca-Cola products in India have been largely overturned after legal actions were filed by the soft drink giant (a few Indian states still outlaw the stuff). Massive advertising and PR campaigns seem to be working, as sales are up 21 percent in India. Coke says the poisons are now gone, but they have played and won this game many times before.

Surviving Coke's "Secret Ingredients"

For those of you who may not know it, Coca-Cola was originally named after

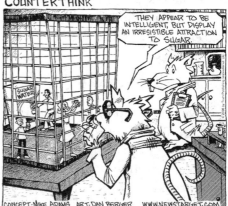

COUNTERTHINK

THEY APPEAR TO BE INTELLIGENT, BUT DISPLAY AN IRRESISTIBLE ATTRACTION TO SUGAR.

CONCEPT-MIKE ADAMS   ART-DAN BERGER   WWW.NEWSTARGET.COM

the addictive drug cocaine, derived from the coca plant, which was added to the original product to induce addiction in children and adults. When the drug was banned, the company replaced it with a slightly less addictive but related chemical, caffeine, extracted from coffee beans. They also added high-fructose corn syrup, which may prove to be the most addictive and toxic "secret ingredient" of all. Coca-Cola is not the only offender. The truth is, all major soft drinks today (Pepsi, Mountain Dew, Dr. Pepper, etc.) are based on a formula similar to Coke's.

No Worries: Healthy Coke

Have you heard about one of the more recent developments in the last few years at the Coca-Cola research labs? Healthy Coke! That's right. Coca-Cola's chief executive at the time it was introduced, E. Neville Isdell, said that his company's new vitamin-enriched cola, Coke Plus, should be included in the health and wellness section of all major 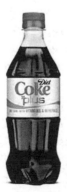 grocery stores. They would like us to believe that Diet Coke + vitamins = a healthy drink. Now you can be healthy and drink Coke too. Ridiculous? Healthy Coke may seem like an oxymoron, but many people are eagerly buying it. Look for it in the health and wellness section at your local grocery store.

Falling for Fake Sugar

The damage to one's health is not avoided by switching to diet drinks. Yes, even today's artificially sweetened sodas and foods are a major problem. They fool your body into thinking that it's actually getting sugar when it's not. This can make your body crave sugar even more. Fake sweeteners are really sweet—160 to 13,000 times sweeter than sugar, making it hard to taste naturally sweetened foods after you've become used to the fake stuff. Have you ever tasted something so sweet and rich that it repulsed your taste buds? What did you do? You probably set it back down. Fake sweeteners dumb down your taste buds' ability to tell you when something is too sweet and much too fattening for you to be eating. Take away this "way too sweet" sensor, and we would eat just about anything. We wouldn't know when to stop.

Although the infallible FDA has approved NutraSweet, Equal, Splenda, Sweet'N Low, Neotame, and other artificial sweeteners as safe for consumption, most of these supersweet, synthetic creations were born in a lab. They don't naturally break down in the body, and they haven't been around long enough for us to determine how they affect humans.

Stick to Grandmom's Honey

If you have a sweet tooth, like I do, it's best to stick with Grandmom on this one. If I want to sweeten something up, I use organic, wild, dark, raw honey. It's not only sweet, but it boosts the immune system, kills unfriendly bacteria, protects teeth and gums from decay, and even helps fight cancer. Let's see the fake sugars do that.

Another alternative to sugar is stevia, a sweet-tasting, nontoxic plant. As a sugar substitute, it has no calories, lowers fat absorption and blood pressure, and because it does not affect blood sugar it is safe for diabetics. Since the 1970s, Japan has been using stevia to sweeten food products like ice cream, pastries, candies, soft drinks, and chewing gum. Today as much as 50 percent of the sweetened products consumed in Japan are made with stevia.

You can also look for foods sweetened with fruit juices and natural cane sugar. These still contain sugar, but in a less processed form, so you get some of the nutrients and vitamins along with the sugar. Don't use brown sugar; it's just white sugar colored with molasses to make it look more natural and less processed. Don't be fooled!

Slow (Food) Poisoning

Did you know someone might be poisoning you? If you are eating nonor-ganic foods, then you are probably eating poisons. Why are there poisons in our food, and how did they get there? You might want to make sure you are sitting down for this one. It all began in 1939, when a Swiss chemist, Paul Müller, discovered the first widely used, synthetically created pesticide. It was dichlorodiphenyltrichloroethane, or DDT. (If you can't pronounce a chemical, it's probably not good for you.) Until the 1960s it was considered a miracle chemical because it could kill a wide range of insect pests but seemed to have low impact on mammals. It didn't break down quickly in the environment, so it didn't have to be reapplied often, and rain didn't easily wash it off plants.

Nobel Pesticide Prize

DDT was inexpensive and easy to apply, and for his discovery, Müller was awarded a Nobel Prize in Physiology or Medicine in 1948. Our government quickly approved its use, and big food companies had a new way to inexpensively kill pests to boost crop yields and make even more money. It was also used as a poison to kill our enemies in World War II.

DDT caught on like a wildfire that spread all over the planet. In 1962 data demonstrated that DDT was a killer, but because it was making so many companies so much money, it wasn't until 1972, some ten years later, that it was declared to be poisonous and deadly to just about every form of life on Earth. It was banned forever in the United States, though many countries still use it.

Tell me again why we should trust the government, the FDA, the Environmental Protection Agency, or the giant food manufacturers with the food we put into our mouths or the mouths of our children, and ultimately with our own Self-Health?

At the time of the writing of this book, 250 basic chemicals made by more than fifty companies are registered for use as pesticides in food and feed production in the United States. Fertilizers, pesticides, and preservatives being used at this very hour on (and in) the foods we buy every day at our local grocery store, restaurant, or fast-food favorite have been linked to a wide range of serious and often fatal conditions: cancer, leukemia, miscarriages, genetic damage, decreased

CONTAMINATED PRODUCE

A study by the Environmental Working Group analyzed results of nearly 51,000 tests for pesticides on fruits and vegetables conducted by the USDA and the FDA between 2000 and 2005. Contamination levels were measured in six different ways and crops were ranked on a composite score from all categories. Below are the foods listed by overall rank, worst to best, along with the results of two of the six criteria studied.

Rank	Produce	Percentage of samples tested with detectable pesticides	Maximum number of pesticides found on a single sample
1	Peaches	96.6%	9
2	Apples	93.6%	9
3	Sweet bell peppers	81.5%	11
4	Celery	94.1%	9
5	Nectarines	97.3%	7
6	Strawberries	92.3%	8
7	Cherries	91.4%	7
8	Lettuce	68.2%	9
9	Grapes, imported	84.2%	8
10	Pears	86.2%	6
11	Spinach	70.0%	6
12	Potatoes	81.0%	4
13	Carrots	81.7%	6
14	Green beans	67.6%	6
15	Hot peppers	55.0%	6
16	Cucumbers	72.5%	6
17	Raspberries	47.9%	6
18	Plums	74.0%	4
19	Oranges	85.1%	4
20	Grapes, domestic	60.5%	7

fertility, liver damage, thyroid disorders, diabetes, neuropathy, still births, decreased sperm counts, asthma, and autoimmune disorders (lupus, chronic fatigue, etc.).

Pesticides for Little People

For children, it's an even grimmer picture. They face all these effects, plus the possibility of birth defects, learning disabilities, and behavioral problems. More than a quarter of a million U.S. children ages one to five ingest a combination of twenty different pesticides every day. More than 1 million preschoolers eat at least fifteen pesticides on any given day. Overall, 20 million children age five and under eat an average of eight pesticides every day.

A recent joint study conducted by Emory University, the Centers for Disease Control, and the University of Washington found that the urine and saliva of children eating a wide variety of regular foods from area groceries, restaurants, and schools contained small amounts of organophosphates, the current family of pesticides spawned by the creation of nerve gas agents in World War II. When the same children ate organic fruits, vegetables, and juices, no sign of pesticide was found.

Interestingly, in the United States it is a violation of federal law to state that the use of pesticides is safe, because pesticides are poison by definition.

These poisons are created to destroy the brains, spinal cords, and nerves of their victims, and yet our government and big food companies encourage our children to swallow these poisons every day (in "safe" amounts, of course). Why? So that big food manufacturers can have higher harvest yields and make more money. There is simply no other reason for it. We let them poison our kids for profit.

For a free, printable, complete list of fruits and vegetables with the highest amount of toxins, check our website, www.SelfHealthRevolution.com.

Pet Food Perversion

If you happen to be a pet owner, don't think for a moment they overlooked your lovable, furry best friend. There are an estimated 55 million dogs and 63 million cats living in American households. That's a lot of pet food and, of course, a lot of money for big food companies. They are not content with just feeding their fake foods to

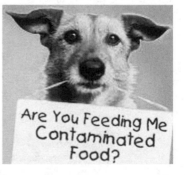

you and your family—they want your pets too.

Before the 1930s, dogs and cats ate mainly what people ate: fresh, organic fruits and vegetables and meats right off the table. But big food companies realized they had to do something with their rejected wheat, rice, and corn that had failed USDA inspection because of rancidity and mold and other contaminants. They also had unwanted and unmarketable meat that failed inspection because it was diseased or spoiled.

Thus the idea of commercial "pet foods" was born—combining two nonconsumable, unusable, rejected foods into a new wonder food for man's best friend. These delicious pet foods are made of what's known in the industry as "4D" meats, that is, meat that is unfit for humans because it's *diseased, disabled, dying,* or *dead* when it arrives at the slaughterhouse. They include "by-products," which is an industry catchall term that means anything from the carcass other than meat itself, such as beaks, feet, heads, lungs, hooves, blood, snouts, and other interesting ingredients.

Preservatives are used in these pet foods as well. Why do you think pet food lasts so long on the shelf? It never seems to go bad, does it? Again, this longevity saves the food manufacturer and the storeowner money, but it's not very good for the pets we love. In fact, one of the most common

pet food preservatives, Monsanto's ethoxyquin, is used not only as a pet food preservative but also as a hardening agent for tires, and it is marked as a poison at their plants (and at those of others storing it) and identified by the Occupational Safety and Health Administration as a hazardous chemical and by the Department of Agriculture as a pesticide (which you know by now means poison). Then there's BHA and BHT, both of which are suspected to cause liver and kidney dysfunction, as well as bladder and stomach cancer. And by the way, all of these preservatives, pesticides, and poisons have been banned for some time in Europe.

Animals with Human Diseases

What are these poisons doing to our pets? We now see very young animals with diseases that used to be seen only in older animals. Many young vets just out of veterinary school think these problems found in younger animals are "normal," but it's definitely a new occurrence. Every day sickly, unhappy dogs and cats arrive in veterinary offices suffering from diarrhea, gas, dandruff, hot spots, vomiting, overshedding, itching, overscratching, face rubbing, foot licking, and chronic illnesses.

Worse still, recent studies have shown that animals that have been forced to join the human fake foods bandwagon by eating pet food are now suffering from human diseases like cancer, arthritis, obesity, dental disease, and heart disease, and they are coming down with these diseases in numbers never seen before. If you are shocked and disheartened by what you have heard about pet food so far, just wait to hear what I have to tell you next.

A Dog-Eat-Dog World

Some pet foods are actually made of pets. I know—it's shocking and seemingly unbelievable. But each year millions of dead dogs and cats are processed along with cows and other animals by big food companies known as renderers. The finished product—tallow and meat meal—is served in pet foods today.

The National Animal Control Association estimates that U.S. animal shelters and veterinarians annually kill 13 million household pets. Thirty percent of these pets are buried, 30 percent are cremated, and 40 percent (about 5.2 million) are sent to rendering factories. When you read "meat or bone meal" on your pet food labels, that means rendered animals, including some dogs and cats. There's no way to really know what animals were used because renderers are not required by law to tell you.

This rendering process has been going on for decades and has been confirmed by numerous federal and state agencies, including the FDA, the American Veterinary Association, and the California Veterinary Medical Association. The government does not control or regulate what kind of animals can or cannot be rendered, so big food renderers and manufacturers simply buy the cheapest carcasses they can find: our pets. As I said, they do this only to make more money. And you thought it couldn't get any worse.

Raise your hand if you're wondering, *Where do I find pet food that won't poison, malnourish, or cannibalize my pet?* Well, if you're a little confused about what pet food to buy, go to our website and you'll get a free comparison list of the most healthful pet foods on the planet. My favorite pet food and the one my dog Polar loves is Castor and Pollux Organix Mix.

Meet Your Meat

We have learned where your pet's food comes from. Now we must turn our attention to the source of our human food. It is time for you to meet your meat. However, let me warn you, it may not be a very pleasant meeting. In fact, what you're about to find out may alter your view of meat forever.

For most of us, our image of cows, chickens, lambs, and pigs is a picture of happiness. We imagine animals

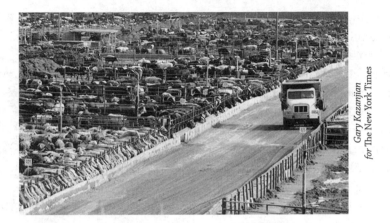

Gary Kazanjian
for The New York Times

strolling through a meadow, chomping on green grass, and enjoying a quiet, peaceful country farm. But that Norman Rockwell view of American farms faded away some forty years ago. The new reality may startle you.

In the 1960s, big food companies began buying small, family-owned livestock farms by the thousands. Most livestock farms today are controlled by only a handful of companies. Instead of having a few hundred animals, like the family farms, these farms have hundreds of thousands and sometimes millions of animals. Instead of letting the animals graze on grass, wander the fields, and bask in the sun, they put them in buildings; feed them corn, among other things (which makes them fat but also sick); give them no room to move; and allow them not one inch of sunlight.

To make these sickly animals even fatter, they inject them with growth hormones and female hormones, and to keep them alive they pump them full of antibiotics. They call these farms "concentrated animal feeding operations." (They can no longer even be called "farms.") I call them concentration camps.

Tortured, Diseased, Stressed, and Insane

As you can imagine, the conditions in these concentration camps are unhealthy, gross, and disgusting. Animals are so crowded that the floor is scarcely visible, and where it is visible, it is covered with excrement and sometimes the carcasses of other animals. Many animals, such as pigs (thought to be as smart as dogs), live their entire life in pens so tight that they cannot turn around, which drives them insane. These animals live unnatural, unearthly, stressed, and tortured lives, directly affecting their immunity, nutrition, and overall health. Can eating such weak, miserable, sick animals have any adverse effect on us?

Why did the big food companies take over these beautiful, family-owned, country farms and create animal concentration camps? One word: efficiency. Think about the new neighborhoods being built today. Remember when houses actually had a yard? It's all about money. More houses per square foot equals more dollars in the bank, and the same is true with farming. What happens when you put animals so tightly together? Simply put, a lot of bad things. For example, what kind of food do you think these concentration camp animals eat? You guessed it: the cheapest possible. Now what I am about to say next may make you sick.

Cannibalism of Cows

If you don't happen to finish your steak at a restaurant, make sure to ask for a to-go bag, or the leftovers might be dinner for a cow (your next steak). It's true. Did you know that calves, instead of drinking their mother's milk, are fed formula made from cows' blood? Yes, this practice is perfectly legal. In fact, the U.S. Food and Drug Administration and the Department of Agriculture allowed cattle to be fed chunks of other cows before the practice was finally banned in 1997 under political

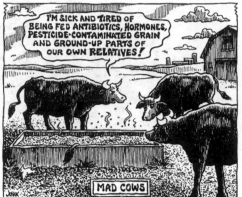

pressure and health fears. The government currently allow cows to be fed chicken litter, leftover restaurant food, and out-of-date pet food. (You already know what that's made of.)

Rendering Changes Everything

Cows are still allowed to eat feed that can include other animals, such as pigs, fish, chickens, horses, even cats and dogs. And some of those animals, before being rendered and mixed up for cattle feed, are raised on food containing the same cow parts now banned from cattle consumption. In order to fatten up, concentration camp cattle continue to consume parts of pigs and horse blood for protein, as well as tallow, which is the fat from rendered cattle parts.

How can the USDA and the FDA allow such practices? Government spokesmen claim that meat that is processed by renderers becomes denatured, meaning it's actually no longer what it was before. So, it is argued, heating the animal parts of dogs, cats, pigs, fish, chickens, and cows to very high temperatures for thirty minutes in the rendering process changes the nature of the meat itself. It is denatured.

In the government's view, the rendered dogs, cats, pigs, fish, chickens, and cows are no longer animal parts, as the rendering process changes them into something called tallow (animal fat) or meat and bone meal (animal protein). It sounds a little like a shell game, where your adversary keeps moving everything around until you can't remember what's true anymore.

Turning herbivores (grass eaters) such as cows into carnivores (meat eaters) and now cannibals (eating their own species) is not only weird and creepy, but has anyone considered what this ungodly experiment is doing to the animals' bodies and the bodies of those humans and other animals that eat their flesh?

Food Fat Farms

The purpose of these concentration camps is to make animals fat. These camps are the true "fat farms," where the more obese you become, the more you are worth. In fact, the USDA rates meat on how much fat it has in it. More fat equals a much higher selling price.

Big food companies do everything they can to make their animals superfat, boost growth rates, and produce more milk, including using growth hormones. (Think cows on steroids.)

Two of these hormones, estradiol and zeranol, are suspected of causing cancer and impacting child development. Female hormones (estrogen) injected in the animals to make them fatter can add an additional forty to fifty pounds to a steer at slaughter. Now many scientists believe that those female hormones find their way not only into our meat but also into our environment. They have been linked to falling sperm counts, premature puberty in young girls, breast growth among men, and sex change (male to female) of fish living downstream from these concentration camps. "Eat meat, get a sex change" might be the motto for these large meat companies in the future.

Cows on Drugs

Concentration camp animals are weak, sick, tired, tortured, diseased, drugged, overmedicated, and undernourished. What keeps these concentration camp animals alive? Ah yes, antibiotics! Of course, this makes the drug companies very happy. Over half of all antibiotics manufactured and sold every year go to concentration camp animals. Yes, animals are given the same antibiotics that humans take. Many fear this could lead directly to the creation of a "superbug," because the more exposure these germs have to antibiotics (whether given to animals or humans), the stronger they become. (Think millions of farm animals.)

Some might say, "Oh, that's okay. It's the antibiotics that keep these poor animals alive." Yes, alive in a system that was created by big food companies to squeeze out every ounce of profit regardless of the cost to these helpless animals or to the creatures who eat them.

What more could they do to our food to make it any worse? Surely, by now they have exhausted every possibility. Well, there is more, and if you're squeamish, you should brace yourself.

Manure in Your Meat

Almost all concentration camp meats found in your favorite restaurant or grocery store have some animal feces on them. Yes, it's true. The butchering process is run at such breakneck speed (to make more money) that when the animals enter the kill floor for slaughter, the feces inevitably spill out and are smeared on the floor. The grinding process quickly spreads this manure from hundreds of different carcasses to millions of hamburgers. Since these feces are likely to contain deadly bacteria like E. coli 0157, the big food com-

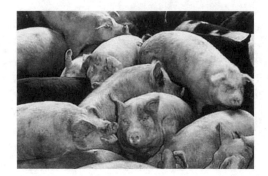

panies concentrate their efforts on sanitizing the feces that will inevitably find their way into your meat by using even more pesticides and low-level radiation.

But don't worry, any feces you might find in your steak or hamburger has been fully sanitized and irradiated for your protection, compliments of your pals at the FDA, USDA, and big food companies.

You Don't Have to Be a Vegetarian

If you love steak and meat, like I do, this news is a big shock and a disappointment. Some of you reading this may wish you never knew what you have just found out. At this point you may want to close your eyes and try to forget about where you now know your meat comes from. But remember, like gravity, the truth is there whether you believe it or not. So don't close your eyes. In the next chapter I will give you alternatives to concentration camp meats that are not only better for the animals but far more healthful for you and full of delicious, natural flavor. If you would like to know right now where to find the best wild-caught, grass-fed, pasture-raised, organic meats in the world, check out our website. This is meat you would like to meet (and eat!).

You Are What You Eat— and What You Eat, Eats Too

The bottom line with fake food is this: Grandmom was right! You are what you eat. In fact, scientists can take fat from your belly, your hips, or your backside, put it under a microscope, and tell exactly where your fat came from. They know whether your fat was formed from eating fat from a cow, pig, lamb, or chicken. Food goes from your lips to your hips, and you become exactly what you eat. And as you now know, what we eat, eats too. That being said, if you were a cow, would you eat you?

If you're eating foods raised in poor soils, bombarded with pesticides, fun- gicides, and preservatives, processed, refined, and depleted of nutrients, then that is what your body is going to be made of. Simple as that. If you are eating obese concentration camp ani- mals that have been weaned on cow's blood, injected with female hormones, medicated with antibiotics, and fed genetically engineered corn, soybeans, cotton seeds, and their own species' fats, laced with slaughterhouse feces and waste, then that is what you will carry around with you in your gut, around your waist, and on your back- side. And it will surely have an effect on your Self-Health.

The Self-Health Dam

A few years ago, a 500-year flood rav- aged the towns and counties of the upper Midwest. Whole city blocks were covered, parked cars were under twelve feet of water, and the govern- ment-constructed levees, dikes, and dams built to protect the people were all failing. Levees that were built by the

> The body is a machine for living. It is organized for that, it is its nature. Let life go on in it, unhindered, and let it defend itself. It will do more than if you paralyze it by encumbering it with remedies.
>
> —LEO TOLSTOY

government to save people were now drowning them.

In the middle of this twice-a-millennium torrent, a few proud, independent folks, knowing the government solution would probably fail, had built their own levees around their homes with their own hands and with their own money. While others lost everything, for these few, their land and homes were high and dry. In fact, in one neighborhood, while everyone else had been evacuated, one such self-dependent owner remained, his house secured by the levee he built himself. He calmly and casually stood with a fishing rod casting into the floodwaters just beyond his front porch, commenting to reporters and rescue crews, "It's a great day for fishing, isn't it?" Now that's Self-Health.

As I said at the beginning of this chapter, each time you sit down to eat, you are making a life-and-death decision. We are indeed digging our graves with our fork and knife. Which food will you find at the end of your fork? Read on, and I will tell you about foods that can make all the difference for your Self-Health and for the health of those you love and care about.

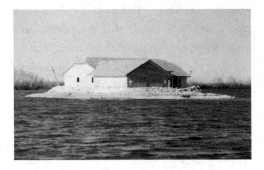

House saved from 500-year flood.

CHAPTER SEVEN

The **Ultimate Brain Doctor**

*What happens one day within the human body is
enough to take away all the luster from fiction.*
—Ralph Waldo Emerson

The human body is the most amazing creation in the universe. From blood circulation (heart, blood, vessels) to digestion (mouth, stomach, intestines), the body has over eleven separate, extremely sophisticated systems, so complex no scientist fully understands them and perhaps never may. The body is made up of over 100 trillion cells (100,000 billion), 206 bones, 600 muscles, and 22 organs. Our eyes can make 10 million different color distinctions, taking in more information than the most powerful telescope. Our ears can discriminate some 1,600 frequencies. Our heart beats 100,000 times a day and pumps blood through a thousand miles of arteries without our even thinking about it.

Can you turn an apple into blood? Your body can. It can change an orange into a kidney, a heart, a liver, or anything it needs, something even the most brilliant team of scientists in the world could never begin to figure out. The body has created and replaced 50,000 cells in the time it took you to read this sentence.

Your Brain Is Your Best Doctor

The human brain, weighing only three pounds, controls all 100 trillion cells in the body. Running on twelve watts, the energy contained in about two large bananas, the brain can store enough information to fill two Empire State Buildings with tiny computer chips fully loaded with data. To date, no com-

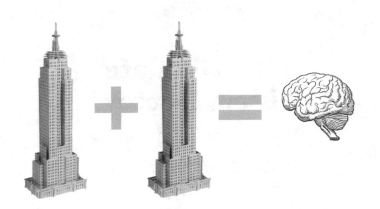

puter or group of computers can equal the overall power of one human brain.

This brain has one overruling goal: to keep your body healthy and alive. That's what it lives for. It works on that single objective twenty-four hours a day, seven days a week. It works while you sleep, while you play, while you eat. It is the most powerful intelligence force in the universe, and it is working for your Self-Health.

Your brain knows more about your individual health than all of the world's doctors, surgeons, specialists, medical centers, universities, researchers, and scientists put together. It's so good at what it does that many of us take it for granted. For instance, notice its amazing work when we cut our finger.

The Miracle Worker

First, the brain sends blood thickeners to the cut to stop the bleeding; then white blood cells are triggered to attack any enemies that might have entered through the cut; it then tells the body to bring a sticky substance, called fibrin, to the location. Fibrin glue seeps throughout the layers of damaged muscle like a web and seals off the wound. The brain then signals fibroblast cells to attach themselves to the injured skin in order to create a bridge to healthy skin. This eventually becomes a scab, which falls off once the wound has healed. All of this happens within a matter of minutes, without our notice or effort, almost miraculously. This same type of healing miracle happens millions of times every day throughout your entire body, healing that goes largely unnoticed.

You're Only Seven Years Old

Your body is a healing machine. It replaces 50,000 dying cells every second and over one billion cells every single day. Your digestive tract is replaced every four days, your immune system every seven days, and most of your body, with the exception of the brain and the eyes, is totally replaced in about seven short years. Whatever your age might be, your body is many years younger: if you are forty, your body is less than ten. (You're younger than you thought.)

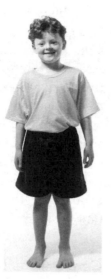

The point is your body is not frail, weak, unintelligent, or vulnerable. If fed the right fuel (living foods), your body is smart, strong, resilient, and capable of unbelievable healing. One of the greatest miracles of the human body is that it finds a way to allow us to survive on the foods we now eat in America.

So if the brain and body are so intelligent and powerful, why are we in America so sick? First, we have to understand what truly causes sickness.

Germs Don't Kill

What comes to mind if I ask, "Where does disease come from?" Germs, viruses, bacteria, or maybe heredity? These are the causes most people think of, and certainly all of these can con-tribute to a specific illness. But are they truly the cause of sickness or disease? Louis Pasteur was one of the first people to see germs under a microscope. He figured out that germs might have something to do with disease, not cursed objects or evil spirits, as was the common wisdom of his day. But there was one thing that he never figured out: Why do some people with these germs in their body never get sick?

Do you know people who never get sick? Maybe you are someone like that. These people can roll on the floor with kids with runny noses, shake the hands of sneezing and coughing coworkers, even have their whole family ill in bed, and they never seem to be phased by all the sickness swirling around them. Somehow they are not vulnerable to the usual germs like the rest of us. Why do you think that is? If these viruses, bacteria, and microbes indeed cause illness, why is this person never affected?

Koch and His Questions

That's the question the Nobel Prize winner and friend of Pasteur, Robert Koch, asked and answered in the previous century. If germs really cause sickness and disease, then why do we sometimes find the disease present in someone's body, but the bug is nowhere to be found? Why do we sometimes find the bug in someone's body, but the disease is nowhere to be

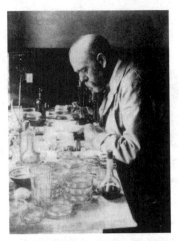

Robert Koch, 1885.

into their throats and on their food. What happened? Nothing. No one got sick. In modern times, the Harvard researcher Andrew Weil has confirmed this. Weil writes, "External objects are never causes of disease, merely agents waiting to cause specific symptoms in susceptible hosts. Rather than warring with diseases with the hope of eliminating them, we ought to worry more about strengthening [the body's] resistance to them."

found? Why can we sometimes take the bug that appears to make someone sick and put it in the body of another person and it does not make that person sick? Why can we take a bug and put it in normal human cells in a petri dish outside the body and it does not make those cells sick?

In one of Koch's experiments, he injected blood from people sick with the flu into sixty-two healthy volunteers. He also sprayed flu germs

Germs Alone Don't Make Us Sick

Weil concluded that germs alone do not cause sickness or disease. These germs can thrive only when our cells are in a weakened state. Normal, healthy cells cannot be affected by germs, bacteria, and viruses outside or inside the body. Many of you reading this book probably have germs in your body right now, yet you are not sick. We are always more likely to get sick when we are tired, run down, not eating right, drinking too much, not sleeping right,

> *All truth passes through three stages.*
> *First, it is ridiculed. Second, it is violently opposed.*
> *Third, it is accepted as being self-evident.*
> —ARTHUR SCHOPENHAUER,
> GERMAN PHILOSOPHER

dehydrated, worried, depressed, or stressed. Isn't that when you get sick? It doesn't take a Nobel Prize winner to figure that out, does it? It's just common sense. (Grandmom already knew this too.)

So if illness and disease do not come from germs, bacteria, and viruses, where do they come from? What's the true cause?

Two Causes of Disease: Malnutrition and Toxins

Almost all illness and disease have two possible causes: malnutrition (eating fake food) and toxins (ingesting poisons). When the 100 trillion cells of your body are being fed living food, clean water, and powerful nutrients, they can function at a level that wards off attacks from all germs, bacteria, and viruses. They simply cannot be defeated. But when the body is fed fake food, depleted of real nutrients, and loaded with poisons, it will fight hard, but eventually it will fail. As I have said before, the greatest testimony to the genius of the human body is its ability to survive the onslaught of fake food that we feed it.

Some people may be thinking, *This is just too simple. I was looking for a much more complex solution. How could a problem so large have such a simple solution?* Would you be surprised if your car didn't run well after I peed in your gas tank? What if I put sawdust in your oil? Better yet, what if I shoved mud up your tailpipe? Would you be shocked if your car didn't crank after such abuse? Our bodies are much more complex and sensitive than our cars.

Flux Capacitor Philosophy

Remember the Flux Capacitor from the popular 1980s movie series *Back to the Future*? Doc Brown, you may recall, originally conceived the idea for the Flux Capacitor on November 5, 1955, when he slipped and hit his head on the sink while standing on the toilet to hang a clock. He envisioned three flashing lights arranged in a Y; according to Doc, this is "what makes time travel possible" for the time-traveling De Lorean DMC-12. All that was needed to power the Flux Capacitor was 1.21 jiggawatts of electricity (not easy to come by). In the second episode Doc Brown pulls into the McFlys' driveway after a trip to the year 2015

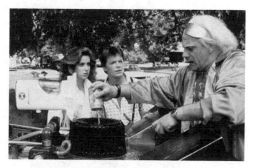

Doc Brown and the Flux Capacitor.

with an attachment called Mr. Fusion Home Energy Reactor, which converts household waste to power. Doc grabs the nearest garbage can and pours its contents and all kinds of random crap into the Flux Capacitor, and off they go.

Many of us see our bodies in much the same way. Food is food is food, right? Just fill 'er up. It will run on anything.

When we put all manner of crap into our system, why are we surprised when our cells struggle, weaken, get sick, and break down? When we give our cells the very best foods, they become strong, full of energy, fit, and powerful.

How are your cells feeling today? Could they use a boost? Would you like to find out more about how to make them feel better? You are about to find out. Are you excited?

CHAPTER EIGHT

Eat Life to Live

The rest of the world lives to eat. . . . I eat to live.
—Socrates

You and I are tiny living beings on a tiny living planet, spinning within a dead massive solar system, hidden within a dead massive galaxy, lost in a universe of billions and billions of dead massive galaxies millions of light years across. As far as we can tell, we are the only living beings in

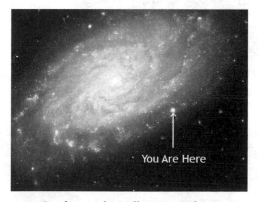

Our home: the Milky Way Galaxy.

the universe. Why are we alive? What gives us life in a universe of death? Three things: air, water, food. If we stop breathing air, drinking water, or eating food, we are dead.

Air, water, and food make it possible for us to exist, and the quality of our existence is based on the quality of these three elements. In other words, the better the quality of the air, water, and food we consume, the better the quality of our Self-Health. If we have rich air, pure water, and living food, we will live longer and live better.

The purity of the air can be quite difficult to control. Good water is a little more accessible today, but it can still be difficult to find. (We will talk more about that later in this book.) On the other hand, food is definitely something that most of us can totally control (believe it or not). As long as our brain guides our arms, hands, and fingers, we can determine what we put in our mouths, can't we? As living beings on a beautiful living planet, what kinds of food do you think we should put into our bodies to feed our living cells? Living food or dead food?

Enzymes: The Force of Life

Is there such a thing as living foods? Of course, there is. Think about it. What kind of food did our great-grandparents eat? Mostly food picked right out of the garden, while it was still alive, before it was cooked, canned, processed, refined, and ultimately killed. Living foods contain the life force of all things in the form of enzymes. Without enzymes, nothing on Earth would exist. Our planet would look like Mars. Enzymes make chemical reactions possible in the world and in your body. There are three thousand known enzymes. They allow you to digest food, breathe, fight disease, see, hear, smell, taste, think, move, and have sex. When the enzymes in your body are gone, you are dead. So enzymes are quite important!

Cooking Kills Life

We have been trained to overcook food. At 118 degrees, all enzymes begin to die. Cooked, processed, refined, canned, and pasteurized foods are all essentially dead foods because the enzymes in them have been destroyed. Much of the American diet today is made up of dead foods. Dead foods are foods that have been altered from their natural state. When we eat dead foods, our body must go into overdrive to produce enzymes from the pancreas to digest those dead foods. This depletes the enzymes the pancreas needs for critical functions like fighting disease.

Great-grandmom got her enzymes from the food she ate, raw living food, so her body did not have to use its own precious enzymes for digestion. Instead her body could use its enzyme resources to fight disease and illness and for healing, repair, and rejuvenation. The reason our generation is so much sicker than Great-grandmom's is that we are all eating mostly dead, cooked, processed food. Cooking and processing food also changes its chemical makeup.

Remember chemistry lab in high school? You poured a compound into a test tube and applied heat to it. What happened? It turned into a totally new compound or substance. The same thing happens to foods that are heated to high temperature. Heating, processing, and refining can change the nature and chemical makeup of food so that it is no longer the same food.

The Good, the Bad, and the Dead

For example, pasteurized milk and raw milk are two uniquely different substances. Pasteurization (a process developed by Louis Pasteur) heats milk to a red-hot 280 degrees, and, yes, it kills all germs, bacteria, and viruses. But it also destroys any good stuff along with it, like enzymes and other nutrients. That's why so many people have allergic reactions to processed, pasteurized milk but not to raw milk. Think about it: most of our great-grandparents drank milk that was fresh from the cow—raw and not pasteurized. They were rarely sick and lived to a ripe old age.

Today much more than milk is pasteurized. Pasteurization is a process we see throughout the food industry, with milk, fruit juices, beer, butter, ice cream, and more. In our rush to kill germs, bacteria, and viruses (none of which can cause illness by themselves alone), we destroy the enzymes and nutrients that our bodies need to have for healthy cells and that will indeed prevent sickness and disease. We have created a sterile food society where neither germs, enzymes, nor nutrients can survive. Now they want to use low-level radiation (irradiation) on our fruits and vegetables for the same reasons.

If you dig a little deeper, you will find that the true motive of the big food companies for the sterilization of our food is actually not consumer protection, but yet another way to preserve and extend the shelf life of their products and once again make more money. (Yes, it's never-ending.) How many products that once lasted only a few hours or days can now be left on the shelf for weeks and months?

If Man Made It, Don't Eat It

Remember Jack LaLanne? He was that fitness guy who, on his seventieth birthday, shackled himself to seventy boats carrying seventy people in the open ocean and swam for a mile and a half pulling the boats behind him. Even in his nineties LaLanne was still in excellent health and worked out two hours every day, an hour in the gym and an hour in the pool. He spent his whole life eating mostly living foods, raw fruits and vegetables. His motto was simple: "If man made it, don't eat it!" He was a guy who truly understood the importance of living foods and Self-Health.

Jack LaLanne had a commonsense approach to eating that has been lost or forgotten over the decades. Once, not that long ago, we were a society of hunter-gatherers. Most of the food we ate (80 percent) was easily gathered from what we planted or harvested wild from the forest. The rest of our food (20 percent) came from hunting,

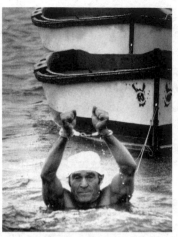

Jack's 70th birthday.

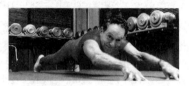

which took great effort with only periodic success. Eating meat in those days was a luxury and a rare treat.

Do you ever watch the *National Geographic* channel? Have you ever noticed how the aboriginal tribes rarely catch or kill anything on their hunts? They usually return to the village with little or nothing and end up eating the plants and fruits that the women had gathered. Meat is a luxury for them. Today, because meat is no longer a luxury for us Americans (thanks to animal concentration camps) and is readily available, we have reversed this equation.

Muscles from Plants?

The average American eats over 200 pounds of meat every year. I grew up thinking I had not eaten a meal unless I had consumed a pretty big piece of meat. If you were raised like me, you might think eating a lot of meat and dairy (proteins) is absolutely necessary for strong bones and muscles. But if you do even a little bit of research, you will quickly discover that this is just not true. Think about it: the biggest animals—gorillas, elephants, rhinos, hippos—all eat predominantly fruits and vegetables. Where did they get the protein to make their muscles so big? I realize our digestive system is designed differently than cows', yet many modern bodybuilders are vegetarians, proving that fruits and vegetables are some of the most powerful, protein-rich foods found anywhere.

All protein is derived from sunlight shining down on plants. Plants absorb the sun's energy and turn it into protein. The cow didn't eat another cow to get its muscles—unless it's from a concentration camp; the cow ate grass. Which food do you think has more protein: 100 calories of sirloin steak or 100 calories of broccoli? If you chose steak, you're wrong. Broccoli has twice as much protein as sirloin steak. Which do you think has more calcium: milk or turnip greens? You probably can guess by now—it's the turnip greens. Nevertheless, we have been programmed to consume large meat portions with very few fruits and vegetables; that's how most Americans eat these days. Could this be the reason we are getting so sick?

Eat Like Poor People

In their groundbreaking book, *The China Study,* called the Grand Prix of all studies of its kind by the *New York Times* (a study involving 130 towns in 65 countries), Thomas and Colin Campbell discovered that when people ate a diet of primarily meat and processed food (dead food), their incidence of cancer and chronic illness increased dramatically. But when they ate a diet of primarily plant foods (living foods), cancer and chronic illness rates fell, and in many cases were virtually nonexistent. In poorer countries, where people invariably eat few animal prod-

ucts, less than 5 percent of the population dies of heart attacks. *The China Study* shows that populations that eat a lifelong diet of mostly plant foods have almost no cancer, heart attacks, and heart disease. In his insightful book, *Eat to Live,* Joel Fuhrman too shows that populations all over the world who get 75 percent of their diet from fruits and vegetables invariably have a much lower rate of killer diseases like cancer and heart disease.

If these reports are true, then cancer, heart disease, and chronic illness are caused by fruit and vegetable deficiency. Get these living foods in your body, and you may not have to worry about dying of one of these diseases.

Eat Like an Aboriginal

In his book, *In Defense of Food,* Michael Pollan discusses a 1982 study of middle-

☐ Percentage of deaths from heart disease and cancer
■ Percentage of calories from unrefined plant foods1

aged Australian Aborigines who had moved near the city and adopted a fake food diet, mainly dead foods like white flour, white sugar, white rice, Cokes, beer, milk, fatty meats, potatoes, and a few fruits and vegetables. They became overweight and diabetic and basically were in poor health. Kerin O'Dea, a nutritionist, convinced the Aborigines to move back to the bush and return to their hunter-gatherer diets (mostly plants, little meat). For seven weeks they ate only plant food, figs, yams, and seafood supplemented with a few wild birds, witchetty grubs, kangaroo, and crocodile.

Seven weeks after they had returned to the bush, O'Dea found stunning improvements in almost every category of their health, from blood pressure to weight (they lost almost 20 pounds each). Even their diabetes was normalizing. What a difference living foods make in our Self-Health.

It may not be practical for us to return to the bush country of our ancestors, but we can still eat like hunter-gatherers by gathering living foods in our very own neighborhood grocery stores. What happens when you start eating more plants (fruits and vegetables)? Until you do it, you can hardly imagine. Living fruits and vegetables are simply some of the most nutritionally powerful foods on the planet. They contain chemicals that can alter your health in a very short time.

The Real Purple Pill

If I told you there was a little purple pill proven to reduce your risk of cancer by a whopping 41 percent (cutting your risk of cancer almost in half), would you take it? How much would you be willing to pay for it? Would you want to share this pill with everyone you love and care about?

According to an article published in the *Journal of the National Cancer Institute* by Jennifer H. Cohen, M.P.H., Ph.D., men who ate three servings of vegetables a week had a 41 percent reduced risk of prostate cancer compared to those who didn't. There's your pill—and you don't even have to visit (or pay) your doctor or pharmacist.

I could spend the rest of this book quoting you study after study showing how fruits and vegetables ward off all kinds of diseases. This may not come as a surprise to you, and it certainly wouldn't surprise our grandparents. What does create skepticism and baffle some people is that plants can also heal. Throughout the ages plants have been known to be agents of healing. From Hippocrates (the father of medicine) in 370 BC to the great Albert Einstein, many people have recognized that fruits, herbs, and vegetables are medicine for our bodies. What is it that makes these plants so powerful? Why are they so good for us?

Oxygen: Friend and Foe

Oxygen is everywhere; the Earth's crust is composed of 50 percent oxygen, the air we breathe contains roughly 21 percent, and 80 percent of all energy production in our bodies is accomplished by oxygen. We can live for forty days without food and seven days without water, but only five minutes without oxygen.

Ironically, although oxygen is necessary for our survival, it actually causes damage to our cells when we use it. When a piece of metal is left out in the weather, in the moist open air, it rusts, right? When you cut an apple in half and leave it sitting out for a while, it turns brown, right? These are both examples of oxidation (rust).

Oxidation also takes place in our bodies. Antioxidants (anti-oxygen) keep things from rusting inside our bodies and protect our cells from breaking down, which leads to aging, sickness, and death. Plants breathe in carbon dioxide and breathe out oxygen. Because plants produce so much oxygen, they need a tremendous amount of antioxidants to protect their own cells. These plant-based chemicals not only prevent the aging and disease (rusting) of our cells, but they also rid our bodies of poisons like pesticides, preservatives, pharmaceuticals, and toxins as well as germs, bacteria, and viruses.

Eat Wide

The greater the number of different fruits and vegetables you eat, the greater the variety of antioxidants and antigerms they will put in your body and the more equipped you will be to fight different varieties of poisons and germs. In the wild, plants are confronted with many enemies: pests, bacteria, virus, and fungus. Over centuries plants have become smart and strong and have developed thousands of chemicals that allow them to fight and win against these enemies. In a world in which every day, more and more varieties of toxins are being dumped, and with all the new germs now evolving, we should be eating more and more varieties of plants. In other words, eat widely.

Plants are chemical-manufacturing marvels. A single tomato has over 10,000 unique plant nutrients, most of which have yet to be fully identified and studied. Just look at the different nutrients and chemicals found in plants that are known to fight disease.

Some Anticancer Chemicals in Plant Food

Allium compounds	Isoflavones	Dithiolethiones
Flavonoids	Polyacetylenes	Liminoids
Phenolic acids	Catechins	Sulforophane
Allyl sulfides	Polyphenols	Ellagic acid
Glucosinolates	Isothiocyanates	Pectins
Phytosterols	Protease inhibitors	Sterols
Anthocyanins	Coumarins	Ferulic acid
Glucosinolates	Lignans	Perillyl alcohol
Caffeic acid	Saponins	Terpenes

This list is only a small sample of the beneficial chemical compounds found in plant foods; new ones are being discovered every day. In the next chapter you will learn some of the most powerful plant foods on the planet. You are about to meet what I like to call the "superfoods."

CHAPTER NINE

Foods Are Medicine

He who does not know food, cannot understand the diseases of man.
Let your food be your medicine and your medicine be your food.
—Hippocrates, the father of medicine, 370 BC

Instead of a drug, picture a super-food, strong enough to fight cancer and heart disease, lower cholesterol, and help you lose weight and increase energy with no side effects. Guess what? These life-altering superfoods are available at your local supermarket just minutes from your home, waiting to be rediscovered.

Broccoli and cauliflower have sulfur compounds that actually destroy cells that go crazy in the body (causing cancer). Broccoli sprouts are ten to one hundred times more powerful than broccoli itself. They fight colon cancer, breast cancer, ulcers, and heart disease.

Blueberries, long part of the Native American diet, are one of the most power-packed, nutrient-dense substances you can put into your body. Their chemicals give blueberries their blue-purple color. The darker the skin of the berry, the more powerful it is. The nutrients in blueberries are known to help lower the risk for heart disease, cancer, diabetes, and Alzheimer's disease, among others. Eat handfuls a day.

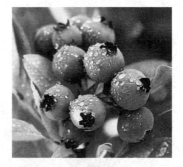

Powerful wild blueberries.

Cilantro is twice as effective as some antibiotics at killing certain types of bacteria and rids the body of heavy metal poisons like mercury. Mercury is an industrial waste often found in water and in many of the animals we eat.

Dried plums contain powerful antioxidants, even more than blueberries. Runners and athletes eat them by the handful before a race to improve their stamina and race time.

Herbs and spices are also powerful. Researchers at the University of Oslo analyzed 1,113 foods to identify those richest in total antioxidants. Of the fifty foods highest in antioxidants, thirteen were herbs and spices. Oregano was found to have forty-two times more antioxidants than apples!

Tomatoes (which in the eighteenth century were thought to be poisonous and to turn blood into acid) contain over 10,000 different nutrients. Lycopene, a potent antioxidant found in the red pigment in plants, is one of those nutrients. Studies suggest that lyco-pene might be a heart saver and that maintaining high levels of lycopene may lower heart disease by up to 50 percent and reduce the risk for tumors.

Popeye knew it! **Spinach** is nature's best source for folate, a B vitamin that prevents birth defects, heart disease, dementia, and colon cancer (the third most common cancer). Another compound in spinach, called lutein, helps prevent macular degeneration, a leading cause of age-related vision loss. Lutein also helps protect skin from the damaging effects of sun exposure; it protects the fats in the top layer of skin, preventing dehydration, roughness, and even wrinkles.

Berries (raspberries, strawberries, blackberries, cranberries, etc.) contain more antioxidant muscle power than any other fruit, strengthening cells against oxidation and inflammation, which are the causes of most age-related illnesses, including diabetes, heart disease, cancer, and Alzheimer's. With a wealth of plant chemicals like ellagic acid, berries reduce tumor risk

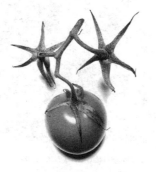

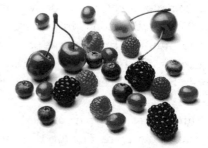

by up to 58 percent, prevent urinary tract infections, increase memory, and help you sleep at night because of a chemical ingredient called melatonin.

Chocolate's botanical name is *cacao*. It comes from the Theobroma tree, which appropriately means "food of the gods." It is said that Moctezuma, the great Aztec emperor, drank forty goblets of hot chocolate every day. Scientists at Tufts University have developed a test that measures the antioxidant power in food, how *powerful* a food actually is, called oxygen radical absorption capacity or ORAC. The cocoa powder in dark chocolate (70 percent or more cacao) outranks just about any food studied when it comes to antioxidants, scoring a 9,000, compared to 2,000 for many other fruits and vegetables. This may explain why dark chocolate lowers the risk for diabetes and hypertension and lowers heart disease by 20 percent by reducing cholesterol and inflammation in the arteries. Chocolate helps keep the arteries young and elastic. Just don't

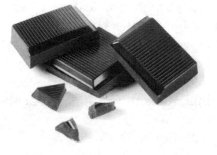

eat too much: the sugar in most chocolates is not good for you.

"Eat your greens!" urged mothers in the 1950s, 1960s, and 1970s. Our ancestors would eat up to six pounds a day of the leafy stuff. It turns out, although it may be irritating to admit, they couldn't have been any wiser. **Dark green, leafy vegetables** like leaf lettuce, romaine, arugula, parsley, chard, mâche, frisée, radicchio, and curly endive are perhaps the most concentrated source of nutrition of any food on the planet. They deliver a powerful punch of minerals (iron, calcium, potassium, magnesium), vitamins (K, C, E, and B), and plant-rich nutrients like lutein, zeaxanthin, beta-carotene, and omega 3's that protect our cells from damage from cancer, heart disease, diabetes, arthritis, and clogging of the arteries.

There is an old Chinese proverb: "Better to be deprived of food for three days, than green tea for one." **Green tea** has been used as medicine in China for at least four thousand years. Now Western science is beginning to catch on. The National Cancer Institute published a study indicating that drinking green tea reduces the risk of certain types of cancer in men and women by nearly 60 percent. Research has shown green tea lowers cholesterol, improves arthritis, decreases the risk for heart disease, fights infection, and improves immune system function.

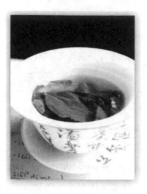

The secret of green teas are their powerful antioxidants. They can kill cancer cells without harming normal cells, and they also inhibit the formation of blood clots that lead to heart attack and stroke. This may explain why the rate of heart disease among Japanese men is so low, even though approximately 75 percent of them smoke.

Why is green tea considered more healthful than other teas? The answer is in how they are processed. Most teas are made from aged or fermented leaves, which changes their health-giving properties, but green teas are steamed, and the steaming keeps all of their original antioxidants intact. White tea is the least processed of all and is the most powerful tea you can drink.

Truth is, all tea comes from the same plant, the *Camellia sinensis*. What typically makes teas different is the length of time their leaves are aged. Aging is the process that makes the leaves turn darker because they are exposed longer to oxygen. White tea, which is picked as a bud, is the least aged; green tea is not aged at all; oolong is semi-aged; and black tea is the most aged of the teas. All of these teas are loaded with antioxidants such as catechins, flavonoids, and polyphenols. Fresh tea leaves (like white and green tea) are high in catechins; the more the tea is aged, the lower the catechin levels. This means that white tea and green tea have the highest levels of catechins, so many people think they are the healthiest. But an interesting thing happens when you age tea: as the catechin level decreases during aging, the level of theaflavins and thearubigins actually increases, so these two substances are found in higher concentrations in oolong and black tea than in green— and yield yet another form of powerful anti-allergy, anti-inflammatory, and anticancer properties.

You can find these teas just about anywhere, but my favorite brand is The Republic of Tea, especially their full-leaf, loose-leaf teas. (Unfiltered brewing is better for you than using teabags.) My current favorite is their powerful, white full-leaf tea called Silver Rain. Another great brand of tea (in bags) is Yumi Tea; it is also 100 percent organic. You can find my special recipe for Kick Tail Tea in chapter 15. I drink three to five cups of tea every day. It gives me a great boost throughout the day.

Aloe vera gel has been recognized for centuries for its healing properties. This strange-looking cactus in the lily family contains an astonishing seventy-five nutrients and two hundred active healing compounds. Most people think of aloe vera only as a skin healer. You may remember your grandmom actually cutting a piece from the plant and applying it to a burn. What many people do not know is that aloe can heal the inside of the body just as well as the outside. Recent studies have shown that aloe juice or gel taken internally can help reduce constipation, diarrhea, indigestion, heartburn, and ulcers, kill germs, and fight disease. I drink aloe vera gel every day in my Self-Health Smoothie. In the smoothie it is tasteless, and it does wonders to heal and preserve the cells inside your body.

Not widely known and certainly underestimated, **clove extract** is derived from an evergreen tree, which produces a flower bud with numerous medicinal properties. It is often referred to as *clove bud*. Clove extract is the most powerful antioxidant ever tested. For example, on the ORAC scale, wild blueberries, thought to be one of the healthiest foods, score about 9,400, but clove extract scores over 10 million. That's the highest score on the ORAC scale to date. A tiny bottle of clove extract is the nutritional equivalent of forty quarts of blueberries. Clove extract aids the digestive process and kills germs, fungus, bacteria, and viruses, fights respiratory illnesses, headaches, stress, and blood impurities, and helps correct sexual dysfunction. I take twenty drops of clove extract every day in my Self-Health Smoothie. My favorite brand is HerbPharm.

To receive a free list of the most powerful fruits, vegetables, and oils ever tested on the ORAC scale, simply go to our website.

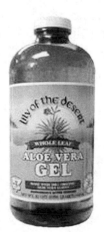

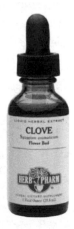

Food That Defends Us

This book does not contain enough pages to print all of the thousands of living foods and plant chemicals and nutrients that can dramatically alter your Self-Health. These living foods have absorbed the wisdom of the universe, and for thousands of generations our human bodies have been utterly dependent on their unique substances for our continued vitality and very survival. There is simply no way around it. We need what they have. Our very DNA demands it. When we don't get it, we become weak, diseased, and sick and we die. To prevent chronic illness, diabetes, heart disease, cancer, and premature death, and to enjoy energy, fitness, health, vitality, and long life, we must find a way to eat, drink, or swallow these precious living foods our bodies desperately need.

In this era, the world has (perhaps unintentionally) conspired against us. From the big food companies that feed us to the physicians we trust, the government agencies we depend on, and the pharmaceutical companies we listen to, I guarantee you, not one of them cares about us like we care about ourselves. For these megabusinesses, in the end it always seems to come down to money and greed. It's time to wake up and realize that no one is going to do it for you.

As strange as it may sound, our best source of defense is the food we choose to put in our mouth. The simple rebellious act that remains within our grasp is to rally against these greedy institutions, defiantly rejecting their Frankenfoods, poisonous prescriptions, and mind-altering advertising, fleeing to the nearest grocery store and stuffing ourselves with the one thing that can truly save us: living foods.

No Health Food Fanatics Here

Have you heard enough? Are you ready for Self-Health? Are you a little nervous about taking the first steps? I understand. So was I. Don't worry, Self-Health will not demand that you stop eating meat. It won't require you

---

It's bizarre that the produce manager is more important to my children's health than the pediatrician.

—MERYL STREEP,
AMERICAN ACTRESS

> *A journey of a thousand miles
> must begin with a single step.*
>
> —LAO TZU,
> THE FOUNDER OF TAOISM

to eat only vegetables or fruits, to give up all of your pet foods and bad habits, become a food fanatic or health nut, stop going to doctors, get off all your pharmaceuticals, stop watching TV, or march on Washington. Self-Health is about waking up from a long deep sleep. It's about slowly opening your eyes and taking baby steps, gradually learning a new way to live for yourself and those you love.

If I asked you to come with me today and run a marathon (twenty-six miles), most of you would tell me that you couldn't possibly do it. But if over the next six months we started walking, then jogging, then running, most of you could indeed (with effort) finish a twenty-six-mile run. That's how Self-Health works. Once your eyes are opened, you want to see more, and the more you learn, the more your beliefs change. And your actions can't help but follow.

Think of something you learned in the past that changed your life. The change was not forced or coerced, but it came naturally, almost without effort, because it was based on your belief, not

on someone else's. When your belief changed, your actions changed too.

Self-Health is not about making massive changes all at once. It is about doing a few new things based on your new beliefs that will dramatically change the health of those 100 trillion cells in your body. Remember, you are building a new body right now (your heart, lungs, liver, kidneys, pancreas, stomach, and skin). Almost all of your cells will be replaced over the next seven years. So what are you going to build this new body with? Let me tell you what you are going to need.

Five Simple Superfoods

There are over two hundred individual nutrients essential to daily, powerful Self-Health. The vast majority of these can easily be found in just five kinds of foods: fruits, enzymes, vegetables, probiotics, and oils (FEVPO). If you can begin to find a way to eat, drink, or swallow these five things every day, you will be well on your way to experiencing increased energy, weight loss, vitality, health, and a long life. I have talked about the first three at length (fruits, vegetables, and enzymes). Now let's spend a few minutes getting acquainted with this dynamic duo: probiotics and oils.

Germs Can Be Your Friends

 I don't want to scare you, but did you know that right now there are over 100 trillion living, breathing bacteria in your gut—three pounds' worth? Over six hundred different species inhabit every normal, healthy bowel, including yours. Disturbing? It certainly can be, especially when bacteria have a reputation for causing disease. However, you need to know that these gut-dwelling good bacteria don't make us sick. In fact, they kill other bad bacteria that do make us sick. They're called *probiotics* (meaning "for life"), as opposed to antibiotics (meaning "against life"), and they work as an extension of your own body's immune system. Think of this bacteria as a hired army that lives in your stomach, working for the brain and body to fight off disease, illness, poisons, and various other enemies (a little gross, but a pretty cool illustration).

One of the bad things about taking antibiotics (besides side effects) is that they kill off most bacteria, including the good guys, the probiotics. In order to kill the bad bacteria that are supposedly causing the disease, we destroy the army of good bacteria that fight for us. That's why antibiotics should be taken with great caution and only as a last resort. Besides, every time you feed bacteria an antibiotic, they learn how to figure it out; it makes them stronger, and they eventually become immune to the antibiotic altogether. Right now in America, and around the world, we are feeding antibiotics to billions of people and animals. (Half of all antibiotics go to nonhumans.) These antibiotics weaken the immune system and kill off the friendly armies of probiotics, while in turn raising up an army of super-strong, super-immune, super-bad bacteria.

An Army of Healers

Clinical studies have shown that these "for life" germs can heal stomach problems (like diarrhea), indigestion, ulcers, allergies, PMS issues, and urinary-tract infections, boost the immune system, maximize nutrient absorption, rid the body of poisons, and kill unfriendly germs. One of their unlikely weapons is an ability to release hydrogen peroxide, which produces an environment in which germs, viruses, and cancer cells cannot live. Remember when you used to put hydrogen peroxide on a cut (long before Neosporin) or gargled with it to rid yourself of a sore throat? These little critters also help break down and remove bad fat (cholesterol) in your small intestines, lowering your risk of heart attack, stroke, and clogging of the arteries.

These powerful and friendly germs are critical to our Self-Health, yet many of us have killed off many of our probiotics, not only by using antibiotics but also by drinking tap water and eating and drinking foods made with tap water, which is loaded with chlorine. Most of us have precious few of the good germs that benefited our grandparents. But don't worry. I will shortly tell you where you can find friendly armies of your own.

Change Your Oil

Have you had an oil change lately? We all know what happens if you don't change the oil in your car. What if you poured the wrong oil into the wrong hole? Choosing to put the wrong oil in your body comes with much more serious consequences than just having to replace you car's engine or buy a new car altogether. The last time I checked, they were not selling new bodies.

Oil is basically melted fat. Our bodies must have fat to function. Fat is as important as protein, carbohydrates, vitamins, water, air, and food. We can't live without it. Fat is not a four-letter word.

In his book *UltraPrevention*, Dr.

Mark Hyman describes a study conducted in 1999 that reveals that we may have received misinformation about fat. For forty-six months, half of a group of 605 heart attack survivors ate a low-fat diet, while the other half ate a diet rich in good fats (fish oil, olive oil, flaxseed oil, eggs). Guess which group did better? The low-fat eaters, right? Actually the folks on the good-fat diet had 50 to 70 percent fewer subsequent heart attacks, while those on the low-fat diet had to leave the study early because too many people in the group were dying of heart attacks.

Know Your Fat

All fats are not created equal. A fat isn't a fat isn't a fat. Some fats are good; some fats are bad. There are basically four kinds of fat: animal fats (saturated fats), plant fats and fish fats (unsaturated fats), and man-made fats (trans or hydrogenated fats). Animals are warm-blooded, so their fat is liquid when warmed to blood temperature but solid at room temperature (think butter). The fat of plants and cold-blooded fish stays liquid at much lower temperatures (think olive oil). Man-made fats do not exist in nature; they were created in a laboratory to make products last longer (and make more money for the producers). Crisco, for example, a fake fat, lasts two years on the shelf, according to their web-

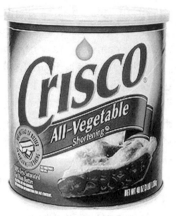

Shelf life of ten years,
say survivalists.

site, but survivalists say it will last for more than ten years. This stuff doesn't break down in your body either. In fact, your body doesn't even know how to digest it. Why does it last so long? Bacteria won't eat it. A good rule of thumb is, "If bacteria won't eat it, you shouldn't, either."

Just about all the fake food from the fast-food giants—McDonald's, Wendy's, Burger King, Jack in the Box, Carl's Jr., Hardees, and Dunkin Donuts—contains some levels of artery-clogging trans fats. Man-made fats are so bad for us that New York and other cities prohibit fast-food restaurants from feeding it to their citizens. (They had to be forced by law to comply.)

Although the FDA allows these food manufacturers to label their products "trans fat free" if the fats are present only in small amounts, these deadly, heart attack–causing fats are found in ordinary foods we know all too well, like Oreos, Orville Redenbacher's popcorn, Quaker Oats, Fruit Loops, Animal Crackers, Fig Newtons, Saltines, fortune cookies (I see heart attacks in your future), and even Girl Scout cookies. Fake fats are approved and sanctioned by the FDA (of course) and are single-handedly responsible for as much as 25 percent of all heart attacks. So be careful to check the label on the processed food you are buying. If you see "shortening" or "partially hydrogenated," it still has trans fat despite the labeling. Yes, it may be within the range that the FDA allows—less than .5 gram—but if you eat three servings of this "trans fat free" food, you could be getting as much as 1.5 grams of trans fat and may be one step closer to a heart attack. Remember Jack LaLanne? "If man made it, don't eat it." If you see trans fats, run away!

Beware of the Big Fat Lie

Labels lie. You know the so-called low-fat 2 percent milk? Well, it's actually not 2 percent fat at all. Thirty-five percent of its calories come from fat. Worse, it's only twenty to thirty calories less than whole milk! They label it "98% fat free" because they measure it by its weight, which includes the water content that contains no calo-

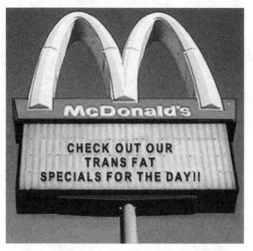

One creative artist's poke at Mickey-D's.

ries at all. It's like mixing a teaspoon of melted butter, which is 100 percent fat, in a glass of hot water, then labeling the glass of melted fat-water "98% fat free." The truth is, water has no calories, and if I were to drink that glass, 100 percent of the calories in it would come from fat. Labels deceive millions of Americans by playing this trick on us with milk, cheese, beef, chicken, and other products. Don't believe their big fat lie!

Alpha and Omega-3's

Among plant and animal fats there are two types: omega-3 and omega-6. Don't worry too much about these space-age names (they refer to the number of atoms in each), just understand that both of these oils are essential for our health.

For millions of years humans ate a diet rich in omega-3 foods, including fish, marine animals, nuts, free-range and grass-fed game, and fresh seaweed. In the early twentieth century, big food companies began dumping cheap soybean oil (containing major omega-6 fats) into the food chain. At the same time we stopped eating as much wild game and fresh fish and began eating concentration camp meats fed on cheaper heavy grains like corn (containing omega-6 fats). As a result, consumption of omega-6 oils has increased a thousand-fold since the early twentieth century, literally changing the cells of our brains and bodies.

Our hunter-gatherer ancestors thrived on an omega-6 to omega-3 oil ratio of 1:1. Some estimates now have the ratio for the average modern American at 40:1. This imbalance and deficiency of omega-3 has been linked to over fifty illnesses, including the dreaded cancer, heart disease, stroke, diabetes, and arthritis.

In 1970 Dr. Jorn Dyerberg, who discovered the benefits of omega-3's, boarded a dog sled and traveled through ice and snow to meet and study Inuit Eskimos. What Dyerberg discovered turned common thinking on its fatty ear. With a diet high in fats (omega-3 oils) and almost no vegetables, fruits, or grains, the Inuit had virtually no high cholesterol, heart disease, cancer, diabetes, or other chronic illnesses. The Inuit could eat the raw blubber (fat) of seals, whales, walruses, and fish and still have one of the lowest death rates from heart disease on the planet, 5 percent, compared with over 40 percent in the United States and elsewhere.

Dyerberg was stunned at his findings and rushed back to report the amazing power of omega-3 oils. Only in the past few years has the very skeptical medical community begun to give credence to what he reported and what the Inuit have known for centuries. Like the Inuit, we should be getting this oil into our bodies in abundance. Don't worry. I won't ask you to eat blubber. These days there are much easier ways to get this miracle oil into your cells. In fact, in the very next chapter I will show you that in just a few minutes every day, you can give your body all the nutrients you need for your Self-Health.

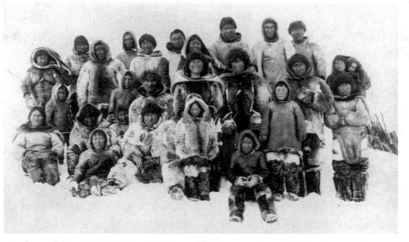

Healthy Inuit village thriving on omega-3 fat.

CHAPTER TEN

Eat, Drink, or **Swallow**

*If I'd known I was going to live so long,
I'd have taken better care of myself.*
—Mickey Mantle, National Baseball Hall of Famer

Now you know the five things you must **eat, drink, or swallow** for your 100 trillion cells to get what they need every day to protect your Self-Health: fruits, enzymes, vegetables, probiotics, and oils (FEVPO). You may be thinking, *How can I do all this? Where do I find the right ingredients? How do I prepare these foods? Is this going to take a lot of time? Is it going to be confusing? Will I like the way this food tastes? Will I have to give up everything I am eating now?* All of these are great questions. Let me tell you what worked for me: the ten-day Self-Health challenge!

Fruits in the Morning

> 1. *Eat fruit every morning for the next ten days.*

Fruits are everywhere: grocery stores, health food stores, farmers markets, maybe even in your own backyard or your neighbor's. It's truly simple. Start eating fruits every morning. Go to the grocery store and pick out your favorites. Make sure you get a wide variety (eat widely) so that you get a broad spectrum of different plant chemicals to feed your cells. There are apples, peaches, plums, cherries, blueberries, blackberries, raspberries, strawberries, kiwis, oranges, grapefruits, watermelon, pears, mangos, bananas, apricots, tangerines, papaya, grapes, and many more.

These fruits are delicious, juicy, and full of energy and nutrients. Start with the ones you like, then venture out and try some new ones. Organic fruits are better for you because they are not raised in depleted soils or with fertilizers, pesticides, and fungicides. (We've already learned what those things do to us.) You can find organics at local health food stores, farmers markets, and now most grocery stores.

If you cannot afford organics or do not live near an organic grocery, don't worry. Start with what you have. Something is always better than nothing. There is a list on our website of the best nonorganic fruits to buy. (Remember, some nonorganic fruits absorb more poisons than others.)

Surround Yourself with Fruit

Stop at the grocery store the night before or on your way to work. Take your Self-Health fruits with you to work. Eat them throughout the morning while others are eating donuts and coffee. Notice how you feel compared to those around you. Once you start eating these fruits every day, you will notice how much better you feel. Soon your body and taste buds will crave these fantastic fruits, desiring these living foods rather than dead foods like bacon, sausage, toast, jam, donuts,

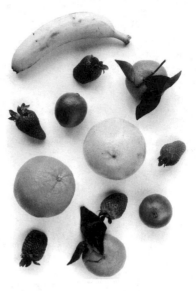

pastries, coffee mochas, bagels, or concentration camp eggs.

While your friends are running to the coffee machine after breakfast because they have no energy, you will just be hitting your stride. You may even find that you're not very hungry come lunchtime. You certainly won't have weakness or fatigue or those distracting stomach growls and cramps that hit you around lunchtime, begging you to fill your face with fake food.

Save yourself now! Eat fruit every morning for the next ten days. Take this challenge, and I promise you will see the difference. In chapter 15 I will tell you a simple, delicious way that I eat my fruit every day (the fifteen-minute Self-Health Smoothie) and give you the easy-to-prepare recipe.

An Enzyme a Day

> 2. *Put enzymes in your mouth every day for ten days.*

Enzymes are the life force of the Earth and our bodies. As you now know, a lack of digestive enzymes can create a boatload of illnesses, including arthritis, obesity, irritable bowel syndrome, heartburn, and chronic fatigue syndrome. When we cook, process, and refine our foods, the enzymes are destroyed. Remember, enzymes are killed at 118 degrees, so the more food you can eat raw or lightly cooked, the more enzymes you are going to get. Try eating raw veggies with your favorite dip or salad dressing. Much of the dressing out there today is not good for you, so try to choose a more healthful one and dip lightly just to get some flavor.

If you don't like raw vegetables, try them lightly steamed. If you're eating out, ask for steamed vegetables. "Lightly cooked or steamed" means the vegetables should still be crunchy. If you are going to eat meat, don't order it well-done—the more cooked it is, the fewer enzymes it has and the harder it will be on your body. You can almost always order steaks and fish medium rare.

A Pill You Should Pop

Even if you eat raw living foods, you will not get all the enzymes your body needs, so you're likely going to need a supplement. Any good health food store should have a good selection of digestive enzymes. Harvey Diamond, the author of *Fit for Life,* one of the top twenty-five bestselling books of all time, has recently come out with his own line of enzymes that are excellent. He even has one that helps digest alcohol and offsets the toxins we get from drinking alcohol. Enzymedica is one of the leading brands and is dedicated solely to enzymes. You can get more information on Harvey Diamond's products and Enzymedica on our website, www.SelfHealthRevolution.com.

You should, of course, talk to your doctor before introducing enzymes or other supplements into your diet. And if you do take them, make sure you choose an enzyme brand that has the greatest variety of active enzymes so that you will cover as many bases as possible. (More is better.) For example,

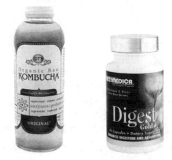

Enzymedica's Digest Gold has thirteen different types of enzymes. You should take these before you eat a meal, especially if you are eating cooked, dead foods. Take them with you to work for lunch and when you go out to a restaurant or to dinner at a friend's house.

A great raw drink that I always have in my fridge is G.T.'s Kombucha. It's part tea, part elixir, and chock-full of enzymes. It tasted a little funky at first, but I have grown to love it. You can find it at Whole Foods Market and any number of health-conscious grocers. For more information, check out our website.

For the next ten days, feed your body enzymes in raw foods, lightly cooked foods, and supplements. I think you will see the difference, and that you will experience much more energy and nutrient absorption, improved digestion (less burping and tooting), and better bathroom experiences. You also won't have to run to the medicine cabinet after meals. Enzymes are the engines of life, so make sure you have them in your body daily as you seize control of your own Self-Health.

Eat Veggies for Lunch and Dinner

> 3. *Feast on veggies for lunch and dinner for the next ten days.*

Eat your veggies! If you're like me and millions of others, when you were lit-

tle you were forced to sit at the table and eat these little colorful enemies (so we thought). No dessert, no playtime, no fun (perhaps even a spanking) until you ate those stupid veggies. Well, if you are still at war with veggies, it's time to make peace. These creations that come in the colors of the rainbow are teeming with life, vitality, and health. Each one can have as many as 10,000 different chemicals and nutrients, including newly discovered anticancer compounds. It won't be hard to find these at your local grocers and farmers markets, and if you're really lucky, you can raise them yourself in your own garden.

You can give yourself the gift of a super Self-Health Salad every day. Pile it high with as many different kinds of greens as you can find (not just iceberg lettuce, please). Start with the ones you know and love and work your way up to those you haven't tried yet.

Remember, variety is the spice of life, and the more veggies you eat, the more likely you are to find the chem-

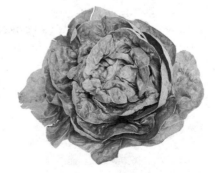

icals your body might be missing. In chapter 15, I will give you my recipe for a fifteen-minute Super Self-Health Salad that I eat every day. It is one of the best-tasting salads you can imagine (awesome reviews so far), and it's one of the most nutritionally potent things you can put in your mouth. "Health in a bowl" is what I like to call it.

Eat the Rainbow

Eat your roots too! Roots are the powerhouses of the vegetable world. The deeper the root vegetable's color, the more antioxidant-loaded plant nutrients it contains. Deep-orange carrots (and black, yellow, and white too) are well known for their beta-carotene (which forms vitamin A); ruby-red beets (and yellow and black also) deliver chemicals good for liver health; purple potatoes are loaded with color pigments that act as antioxidants. In addition to these, there are turnips, yams, sweet potatoes, radishes, potatoes (ten or more kinds), rutabagas, and parsnips, just to name a few. So eat roots and eat the rainbow. I will show you in chapter 15 an easy way to incorporate these color-coded roots into your Super Self-Health Salad.

Variety Is the Spice of Life

The choices are endless! There are so many other fresh, delicious, living veg-gies you can try: asparagus, squash, corn, celery, tomatoes, avocados, broccoli, cauliflower, brussels sprouts, beans, eggplant, cucumbers, mushrooms, okra, peas, cilantro, bell peppers, cabbage, artichokes, and fresh herbs—and I am just getting started. You can cut these veggies up, add them to your Self-Health Salad, steam them, lightly cook them, dip them in your favorite salad dressing or even dark chocolate (at least 70 percent cacao). Have some healthful fun!

If you crave meat, turn your salad into a dinner entrée and throw in some wild-caught salmon, free-range organic chicken, or organic grass-fed beef.

You can eat as much of these types of food as you want and you will not get fat. I dare you to try. You also will not get that bloated feeling of overeating. You know the one, where you wish dinner chairs could be turned into recliners. Eat these vegetables every day for ten days and your body will experience a revolution. You should have more energy than a kid, and you may start to lose weight almost immediately; your body will start craving this food; you will seek out these vegetables at the market, at restaurants, even on the plates of others. (You can score high here, as others may not want their veggies.) You will find that your body no longer has the cravings for junk food it used to.

One reason we overeat, binge, and

become overweight and eventually obese is because our body begs us to keep eating long after our bellies are filled. The fake food we take in has so few nutrients that the brain demands more and more in an effort to satisfy its nutrient needs. Once our body gets the food it needs, it stops begging for more. So take the ten-day Self-Health challenge. Put these wonderful colors of the rainbow into your body and revolutionize your Self-Health.

Probiotics (for Life)

> 4. *Put probiotics in your belly every day for ten days.*

There are six hundred different types of good and bad bacteria in your intestines at any given time. The good bacteria are there to fight the bad bacteria. As you now know, these good bacteria can be hard to find because we kill most of them through chlorinated washes, pesticides, fungicides, preservatives, cooking, pasteurization, and processing. But you can still find these helpful little creatures in a few fermented foods, such as yogurt, miso, sauerkraut, pickled vegetables, kefir, kimchi, sour cream, buttermilk, and cheese. Look for the words "live and active cultures."

Swallow an Army

Once again, because of modern sterilization, most of us will not get enough of these little critters into our body. You should take at least one probiotic supplement every day. Look for brands that have the largest variety of friendly bacteria in them. Remember, more is better. A greater variety means more probiotic armies in your body fighting with different kinds of soldiers to take on different types of enemies. Think general army troops versus Green Berets, Army Rangers, Navy Seals, and Air Force paratroopers, each with a different job to do and very specialized at kicking the enemy's butt. There are a few great probiotic brands to choose from, but I prefer Nature's Way Primadophilus Optima, as they guarantee the quality of their product. Each tablet contains fourteen different probiotic strains. You can find them at Whole Foods Market or your local health food store. You can obtain

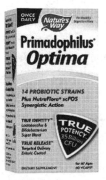

more info on probiotics resources on our website.

Taking these wonderful little probiotics for the next ten days will create troops of friendly bacteria in your tummy. Most people find improved digestion and more pleasant bowel movements and bathroom experiences. Probiotics boost the immune system and clean the digestive tract of toxins. Try them!

Drill Your Own Oil Daily

> 5. *Change your oil every day for the next ten days.*

Some of us who are getting along in years (no names, please) may have traumatic memories of being forced to swallow a spoonful of cod liver oil every day. Torturers they may have been, but it seems Grandmom and Grandad were right on this one too. Once again, after being snubbed by modern medicine, cod liver oil (omega-3 oil) is considered a cure-all for poor memory, cancer, heart disease, stroke, diabetes, and arthritis. Fatty cold water fish such as salmon, mackerel, anchovies, herring, and sardines are great sources of omega-3 oils.

Fish (Food) Coloring

If you do eat fish, you might want to seriously consider buying only wild-caught fish. Most fish sold commercially today (tuna, salmon, catfish, tilapia) is farm-raised in big pens with millions of fish swimming in their own waste. They feed these fish a special fish chow and load them up with antibiotics and hormones. Farmed salmon are fed chemical additives (think food coloring) to make their flesh turn orange so they look like wild-caught salmon. Don't believe me? Check out the fish market at your local grocery store and you will find that unless it's Whole Foods Market, they will have a sign in front of the salmon display that says, "Artificially Colored," which is required by law (the only reason the sign is there).

You can always tell fake salmon (food coloring and all) because its flesh is light orange in color and full of white fat, compared with wild salmon, which is always deep orange, almost red in color, and has very little fat. Can you believe they have even figured out a way to make fish fat?

Don't like fish? That's okay. Flaxseed, flaxseed oil, organic omega-3 eggs, and kiwifruit are nonfishy sources of these good oils. Flaxseeds have nearly six times the omega-3's found in fish. Even more nutty sources (pardon the pun) of omega-3 oils include walnuts, Brazil nuts, hickory nuts, macadamia nuts, almonds, and butternuts. In chapter 15 I'll give you a great recipe for some tasty Self-Health trail mix

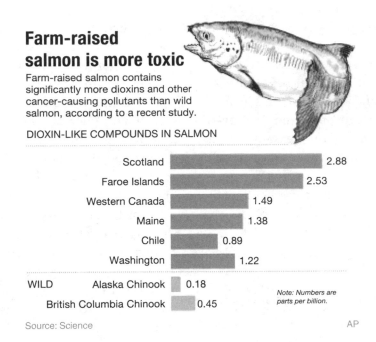

Farm-raised salmon is more toxic

Farm-raised salmon contains significantly more dioxins and other cancer-causing pollutants than wild salmon, according to a recent study.

DIOXIN-LIKE COMPOUNDS IN SALMON

Scotland	2.88
Faroe Islands	2.53
Western Canada	1.49
Maine	1.38
Chile	0.89
Washington	1.22
WILD Alaska Chinook	0.18
British Columbia Chinook	0.45

Note: Numbers are parts per billion.

Source: Science

AP

that combines omega-3 nuts and seeds with dried fruit for a combination that is guaranteed to knock your socks off.

No Fishy Flavor

Although food is the best source of oils, you probably won't eat enough fish or flaxseeds to give your body the oil changes it needs on a regular basis. At your local health food store you can find flaxseed and fish oil in liquid and pill form. You can put the liquid in your Self-Health Smoothie and not even notice it's there (I promise).

For fish oil or cod liver oil the only brands I trust and personally use are Nordic Naturals and New Chapter Wholemega. There is more info on these brands on our website. These brands source their fish from pristine waters, harvest their fish the same day they are caught (which ensures freshness), and routinely check their fish for poisons like mercury (a nervous system poison), which is being found in heavy amounts in the fish population due to pollution.

For the next ten days get this healthful omega-3 oil in your body. You may begin to see improvements

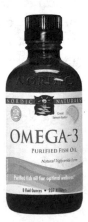

in your memory and feel calmer, less stressed, and more positive about life. Your brain is 60 percent oil (fat), and omega-3's are one of the most powerful foods you can feed it. In a pill or in a smoothie, change your oil and change your life. Try it for ten days and see if it works. I dare you to see the difference.

Back Up Your Food

No matter how much awesome living food you consume, you may find that you are missing some distinct micronutrients that are not available in the varieties of foods you are eating. For this reason, I back up my food with at least a few supplements, such as a whole food–based multivitamin and a robust greens powder. My favorite multivitamin is MegaFood because they use a low-heat process and have the best sourcing, followed by New Chapter and Garden of Life. The greens

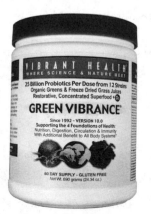

supplement I use every day is Green Vibrance. It's packed with hundreds of plant nutrients you probably will never see in your diet. There's more info on supplements that back up your food on our website.

The D3 Dilemma

There is one vitamin that we need in amounts twenty-five times what the government currently recommends, and 70 percent of us are probably not getting enough. This all according to a recent study by Dr. Michael Holick from Boston University Medical School.

This same vitamin has disappeared from our food supply, and its absence has recently been linked to heart disease, high blood pressure, diabetes, cancer, muscle pain, bone loss, and many other illnesses. What is this incredibly important missing nutrient? Vitamin D3.

Vitamin D3 puts your body's cells into an anticancer state by reducing cellular growth and regulating genes, which explains why D3 deficiency has been linked to breast, ovarian, colon, and prostate cancers. Our bodies manufacture D3 when we walk out of our buildings and cubicles and into the beautiful sunlight. In fact, 80 percent of the D3 we need comes from the sun. When our skin turns slightly red from sun exposure, it means our bodies are getting at least 10,000 units of D3. The problem is we are not out in the sun as much as we used to be, and when we are, sun block, while protecting against skin cancer, also blocks out the D3 our bodies desperately need.

So how do we get more D3? You can start by eating more wild salmon, mackerel, sardines, free-range organic eggs, and fish liver oils such as cod liver oil (which is tasteless in your Self-Health Smoothie). But still you may not be able to eat enough food to give you the 2,000 International Units (IUs) of D3 recommended by the brilliant vitamin D pioneer, Dr. Holick, professor at Boston University School of Medicine. I personally take at least one Carlson's D3 4,000 IU supplement every single day.

You Eat What You Put on Your Skin

Skin is the largest organ of the body. More than 60 percent of whatever you put on your skin gets directly absorbed into your body, just like the nicotine patch people use to help them quit smoking. You simply put on the patch and your skin begins sucking in small quantities of nicotine, which enters your blood and eventually becomes part of your body tissues. In the same way, you are slowly eating whatever you put on your skin. If it goes on your skin, it winds up in your body.

Many of the products we put on our skin, such as moisturizing lotions, deodorants, shaving creams, cosmetics, insect repellents, sunscreens, and colognes and perfumes, are so poisonous that if you put them in your mouth you would immediately become very ill and possibly even die. That's why our friends at the FDA have determined that many chemicals are for external use only. They are poisonous and cannot be taken internally because they can kill you. Yet, ironically, they allow us to put these same chemicals on our skin. Hmm . . . is the FDA really this stupid? (This sounds like a George McFly moment from the movie *Back to the Future*.) These toxic substances date as far back as 1938, when the very first consumer products laws were enacted. Major companies continue to use the same formulas from sixty years ago because they sell better and are much cheaper to produce. Cosmetics manufacturers wield a great deal of influence at the FDA through lobbyists and politicians in order to keep their original formulas and keep profits high.

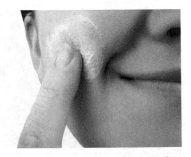

Sixty percent is absorbed on skin.

Antifreeze Skin Care

Would you drink a glass of antifreeze? Or rub it all over your body? How about putting a little engine degreaser in your hair? If you are currently using over-the-counter cosmetics and shampoos, you probably already are. Two of the three ingredients in antifreeze are glycol-based, and glycol and its derivatives are in most skin care and personal care products today. Take a look for yourself. Grab a bottle of your favorite shampoo, lotion, soap, or cleanser. Look for the whole family of glycols: propylene glycol, butylene glycol, polyethylene glycol, and ethylene glycol. These are petroleum derivatives that act as solvents (think engine degreaser), and they can easily penetrate the skin. In fact, glycols penetrate the skin so quickly that the Environmental Protection Agency warns factory workers to avoid skin contact to prevent brain, liver, and kidney abnormalities.

There are other poisons you might find lurking in your cosmetics. The following list is from Len and Vicki Saputo's revealing book, *A Return to Healing.*

Mineral oil, paraffin, and petrolatum: Petroleum products coat the skin like plastic, clogging pores and creating a buildup of toxins, which in turn accumulate and can lead to dermatologic issues. They slow cellular development, which can cause much earlier signs of aging. They are a suspected cause of cancer and also disruptive of normal hormonal activity. Why do you think that when there's an oil (petroleum) spill in the ocean, they rush to clean it up?

Parabens: An estimated 13,200 cosmetic and skin care products (including moisturizers) contain parabens. They have hormone-disrupting qualities, mimicking estrogen; interfere with the body's endocrine system; and are implicated in the occurrence of cancer.

Phenol carbolic acid: Found in many lotions and skin creams, these can cause circulatory collapse, paralysis, convulsions, coma, and even death from respiratory failure.

Acrylamide: Found in many hand and face creams, it is linked to mammary tumors in lab research.

Sodium lauryl sulfate (SLS) and sodium lauryl ether sulfate (SLES): Found in car washes, engine degreasers, garage floor cleaners, and in over 90 percent of personal care products, SLS breaks down the skin's moisture barrier, easily penetrates the skin, and allows other chemicals to easily penetrate the skin. Combined with other chemicals, SLS becomes a nitrosamine, a potent class of carcinogen. It can also cause hair loss. SLES is sometimes disguised with the labeling "comes from coconut" or "coconut-derived."

Toluene: Poison! Danger! Harmful

or fatal if swallowed! Harmful if inhaled or absorbed through the skin! Made from petroleum or coal tar, toluene is found in most synthetic fragrances. Chronic exposure is linked to anemia, lowered blood cell count, and liver and kidney damage, and may affect a developing fetus. Butylated hydroxytoluene (BHT) contains toluene. Other names are benzoic acid and benzyl.

Dioxane: This chemical is found in compounds known as PEG: polysorbates, laureth, and ethoxylated alcohols. Dioxane's carcinogenicity was first reported in 1965 and later confirmed in studies, including one from the National Cancer Institute in 1978. Nasal passages and the liver are the most vulnerable. A 1992 FDA survey found this highly toxic chemical in twenty-seven out of thirty children's bubble bath and shampoo products. It is a synthetic derivative of coconut, so watch for hidden language on labels, such as "comes from coconut."

For more information on toxins in cosmetics, see our website, where you will also find a complete, printable list. A good book to read is *The Safe Shoppers Bible*, published in 1995, by Dr. Samuel Epstein and Dr. David Steinman.

Feed Your Skin from the Outside In

What kind of nutrients would you like to have inside your body? Put those

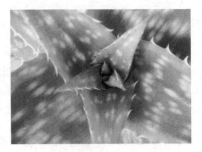

The healing aloe plant.

same ingredients on your skin, and you will also put them into your body. One of my favorite things to put on my skin and in my body is aloe vera. It has been recognized for centuries for its remarkable healing properties. A single aloe leaf contains at least 75 nutrients, 200 active compounds, 12 unique minerals, 20 of the 22 necessary amino acids, and 12 different vitamins.

The following are some other powerful plants to put on your skin and in your body. The list is from Susan West Kurz's enlightening book *Awakening Beauty the Dr. Hauschka Way*.

Lavender is one of the most effective and widely used herbs in skincare and healing. It is an anti-inflammatory, an antispasmodic, and an antiseptic.

Chamomile relaxes muscles, connective tissues, and the skin itself. It is also a great immune booster and is frequently used to enhance liver and digestive function.

Rosemary originated in the Mediterranean and is a lover of sunshine, which the plant captures in its tiny leaves and retains in its essential oils. Rosemary is traditionally used to treat abdominal pain, colic, gout, rheumatism, chronic weakness, and low blood pressure.

Lemon is used in Chinese medicine to cleanse and heal the liver and promote digestion and stronger bowel elimination. It is used by the cosmetics industry because it contains alpha hydroxy acids, which reduce and prevent wrinkles.

Witch hazel is an anti-inflammatory and has potent antioxidant powers. It is traditionally used to treat diarrhea and inflammation of the gums and mouth; to promote the healing of wounds, hemorrhoids, and varicose veins; and as a topical salve for all types of skin disorders.

Saint-John's-wort is most recognized as an herb that can relieve mild to moderate depression. Its essential oils are rich in antioxidants. Taken internally or applied directly, it can heal and close large pores and openings on the skin. It relieves pain, promotes healing of the skin and other tissues, and calms the nervous system. Saint-John's-wort is used by herbalists and homeopaths to treat all kinds of skin disorders, including chapped, cracked, or irritated skin, acne, and mild burns.

The **anthyllis flower** promotes urinary and kidney health. Traditional herbalists in Europe used anthyllis to heal wounds and treat skin disorders of all types, including acne, rosacea, dermatitis, and skin rashes.

The **bryophyllum plant** is an excellent moisturizer. It rejuvenates the skin while stimulating it to retain its own moisture. It also contains many healing chemicals, including calcium and flavonoids. It is highly anti-inflammatory and immune boosting and promotes wound healing. As it moisturizes, it also heals and restores the skin's flexibility, durability, and firmness.

The **calendula flower** was discovered by ancient healers who observed that it bloomed each day at approximately 9 a.m. and closed its petals at 3 p.m., with the rising and setting of the sun. In this way the calendula flower could absorb and retain the potent healing energies of the sun. The calendula is loaded with powerful healing substances, including essential oils, saponins, carotenoids, and flavonoids (all plant nutrients). It has been used throughout Europe to heal wounds, reduce inflammation, and treat bruises, burns, cuts, and skin ulcers.

These are only a few of the nutrient-rich plants for your skin to eat. You can find many more in the body care section of your local health food store. Make sure you look for organic, biodynamic products. I use these products for toothpaste, mouthwash, shampoo, shaving, deodorant, lip balm, and lotion. Some of my favorite brands are

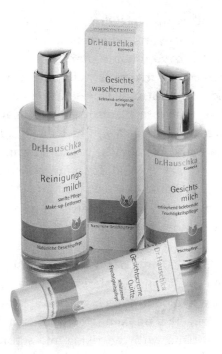

Dr. Hauschka skin care, John Masters hair care, and Aveda Organic products. Don't forget to always read the label and look for the good stuff and avoid the bad stuff. Remember, you are what your skin eats too.

Red, Red, Wine

Grape skins and seeds contain resveratrol, a substance considered by many to be the true anti-aging chemical. This powerful plant nutrient can heal skin, reverse aging, prevent heart disease, and fight cancer. Resveratrol is found in large amounts among grape varieties, primarily in their skins and seeds, which, in muscadine grapes, have about one hundred times higher concentration of this powerful chemical.

You can't really talk about resveratrol these days without at least commenting on red wine. There does seem to be supporting evidence that a glass or two of red wine a day can be good for your health. The fact is, if you are going to drink at all, you probably should be drinking only red wine.

One question I am often asked is "Which grapes have the most resveratrol?" Resveratrol is the "antibiotic" that grapes make when they're under attack by pests, diseases, or fungus. So the wine grapes with the most resveratrol are those grown in northern climates (cool, wet weather) and grown organically (have to fight to survive). In a study of hundreds of wines from around the globe, the Cornell researcher Leroy Creasy found the highest resveratrol levels in pinot noir grapes, probably due to their sensitivity to fungus and bacteria (only the strong survive).

However, Roger Corder, in his book *The Red Wine Diet*, deduced that OPCs, or anthocyanins (strong antioxidants), not resveratrol, were the reason for wine's health benefits. He points out that the people of southern France live longer and drink only local Madi-

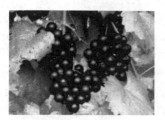

Muscadines 100x resveratrol.

ran wines, made with Tannat grapes, which have the highest concentration of OPCs of any grape. Whatever the case may be, if you're going to drink, organic red wine is your best Self-Health bet. Of course, if you can find it, wild Muscadine wine would be my first choice. You might even catch me sipping a glass from time to time.

Is Eating Out Eating Out You?

Eating out may be eating out your stomach, your liver, your heart, and your lungs. Because of our busy schedules, many of us find ourselves eating out several times a week; some of us eat out almost every meal. Restaurant food is some of the most processed food you can put in your mouth. The commercial fake food arrives in big-food company trucks (90 percent of all restaurants get virtually the same food) and is lovingly prepared using can openers and microwaves. If you're counting on restaurants to promote your Self-Health, you are making a serious miscalculation. But everybody eats out (including

me four or five times weekly), so what do you do?

First, you have to plan on getting your Self-Health somewhere other than the restaurant kitchen. If you are drinking your Self-Health Smoothie and eating your Self-Health Salad once or twice a day, then you are giving your body most of what it needs. Even if you are going to eat out for lunch or supper, give your body what it needs first. If you do, then you won't eat nearly as much commercial cooking at the restaurant. Second, seek out cafés and restaurants that prepare organic, heirloom, homemade, nonprocessed foods. More and more of them pop up all the time. Whole Foods has a wonderful café and food bar; many other health food stores also have restaurants attached. Third, look for living foods on the menu like raw or steamed veggies, fresh fruits, organic, wild-caught fish, and free-range beef and chicken. Order your fish and red meat cooked medium or medium rare because it will have more enzymes and nutrients.

The bottom line is this: Don't rely on eating out for your Self-Health! Get your living food before or after you go to the restaurant. It will take a little effort and planning, but it's much more convenient than diabetes, open-heart surgery, radiation therapy, or chemotherapy. It's your life, and if you don't protect it, no one else will.

Too Poor for Produce?

Some of you may be thinking, *All this wonderful food and nutrients in my body for the next ten days really sounds wonderful, but how in the world will I ever pay for it? In this economy, I am barely getting by as it is. Now you're asking me to spend even more?*

Believe me, I do understand why you might feel this way. In fact, I thought the same thing when I first got started. I come from pretty humble origins; my family worked hard for every dollar. I clearly remember times my mother and father had to struggle to figure out how to keep enough food on the table. That said, buying healthful food may not cost you as much as you think (only 20 to 30 percent more). Here's why.

Less Food Is More Food

Remember, one reason we suffer from food cravings and binges is because our bodies are literally starving for more nutrients. Cheaper, processed, fake foods are stripped and sucked dry of these necessary nutrients. In an attempt to make up for this emptiness, our bodies must consume massive volumes of fake foods. Think about the humongous portions served to us at our local restaurants, cafés, and diners, not to mention all-you-can-eat buffets. Portion sizes across the board

are exponentially larger than they were only twenty years ago (bigger portions, bigger profits, bigger people). Even our plates at home have gotten larger, from your grandmother's nine-inch plates in the 1950s to over twelve inches today. And they're still growing.

When living the Self-Health lifestyle, you are consuming much more powerful, nutrient-dense foods, so your body is not forced to eat quite as much in order to feel satisfied. This may not seem possible at first, but you will see that it does work. (Just as better fuel takes your car farther.) And less food equals less money spent at the market. So your food costs a little more, but it goes a lot further. And you're going to love how it makes you feel (no more bloating after dinner). Plus, serving your meals on smaller, ten-inch plates can save you about 20 percent on your caloric intake and about 10 pounds a year off your waistline.

Home Is Where Your Heart Lives

These days only half of what we eat is food we make ourselves; the other half is mostly defrosted, microwaved, and reheated food we consume from fast-food and sit-down restuarants (much of it from the same food trucks that stock most restaurants). If you really want to save your family's Self-Health, determine now to start preparing and eating more food at home (more like 75 percent). Kids alone consume 55 percent more calories when eating out, compared to eating foods prepared at home. You may be thinking this is a good idea in theory, but impossible to achieve with our busy schedules. I truly understand, but you always have time for what's really important to you. Here are a few time-saving tips that work well for me.

When I'm in a hurry, I simply bypass the fast-food joints and head straight to my local grocery store, where I can usually find a beautiful hormone- and antibiotic-free, cooked rotisserie chicken for around $7 (organic is $9). I simply add my favorite vegetables and maybe some brown rice. Presto, I have a delicious, healthful meal. Health-conscious groceries now also offer drug-free and organic, prepared beef, fish, turkey, and pork. You can pick it up, run home, and mix it with your favorite veggies and whole grains. Many health-minded grocers are now offering family meal deals that feed four people for around $15 to $20. Eating at home can be much easier and much more affordable than you realize! Plus, you might actually get some qual-

ity time with your family members. For more ideas on fast, healthful meals you can make quickly, check out our website.

Don't Let Organics Stop You

If you can't afford the more expensive organic, grass-fed, wild-caught foods, then don't buy them! Buy what you can afford. You can still buy nonprocessed foods, conventional fruits and vegetables, whole grain breads and rice, and steroid- and hormone-free meats. You'll still be so much better off by putting this stuff in your body, even if it's not all organic. Some foods have more toxins than others. There's a comparison list on page 53 and a more complete list on our website that you can print out.

The important thing is that you start feeding yourself and those you love the most healthful foods that you can afford. So please don't let the price of organics be an excuse for you not to join the Self-Health Revolution. Get out there and get the best nutrient-dense foods you can afford.

Pay the farmer now or pay the doctor later.
—OLD AGRARIAN PROVERB

Pay Now, Live Later

In 1970 we spent 20 percent of our income on food. With the advent of mass-produced fake foods, we now spend only 10 percent, and it's going even lower. (Perhaps McDonald's will end up with a 50 cent menu.) We are now learning the hard way that, when it comes to food, you get what you pay for. It may be time for us to put our money where our mouth is and decide to eat to live.

Decide right now that your and your family's Self-Health is worth an extra 20 to 30 percent in your food budget. If you or someone you love is diagnosed with heart disease, cancer, or another chronic illness, it's going to cost you much more in money, time, and lifestyle. If you start now, eating fewer calories by choosing powerful, nutrient-dense foods for your meals, you can actually lower your grocery costs. If you reduce your expenses by avoiding the top four things typically purchased in grocery stores (sugar, caffeine, nicotine, and alcohol), you will certainly decrease your budget. If you buy your food from local farmers and farmers markets, you can often save big on produce and get more healthful foods into your body.

Sometimes making the Self-Health transition is not always about time or money. Your family, friends, spouse, and children may initially resist the Self-Health change. That's very normal and to be expected. All change happens in the mind. Have them read my book or, if they won't read it, read portions of it to them. Slowly start to mix the

Self-Health Summary: The Ten-Day Challenge

5 Things Your Body Must Have Every Day (from chapter 10)

FEVPO =   **F**ruits   (Eat widely)
                Enzymes   (Broad spectrum)
                Vegetables   (Eat widely)
                Probiotics   (Broad spectrum)
                Oils   (Pristine source)

2 Things You Must Eat Every Day to Get FEVPO (from chapter 10)

- 15-Minute Self-Health Smoothie (recipe in chapter 15)
- 15-Minute Self-Health Salad (recipe in chapter 15)

Self-Health Salad, Smoothie, and other wonderful foods into their diet. Their bodies will start craving these powerful nutrients, and over time they will want more. Like anything in life that is truly valuable, it will take time and effort, but the outcome is indeed worth it. Picture the people you love living healthy, long, energetic lives, free of chronic illness, debilitating disease and pain. What's that worth to you?

CHAPTER ELEVEN

Living Water and Air

Fresh air, water, and food impoverishes the doctor.
—Danish proverb

Over the next ten days you are going to give yourself the awesome gift of living foods, which will truly revolutionize your life. Just as important, over the next ten days, it is crucial that you give yourself the gift of living water. Water is the basis of life.

Although over 70 percent of the Earth's surface is water, 98 percent of it is saltwater. Only 2 percent of the Earth's water is drinkable, fresh water, and the majority of this is trapped in frozen ice and glaciers. Seventy percent of our body is made up of water. And like the Earth, our body is also made up of salt and fresh water (like having two oceans inside us). The water inside our cells is fresh water, and the water outside our cells is salty.

Water is clearly a basic ingredient of your body's chemistry. The bones that frame your body are 25 percent water, the muscles that move your body are 75 percent water, the lungs that breathe oxygen for your body are 90 percent water, the blood that carries

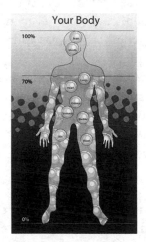

Your Body

100%

70%

0%

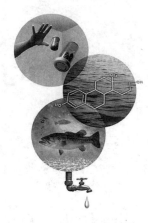

nutrients throughout your body is 82 percent water, and the brain that controls all of your 100 trillion cells is made up of 76 percent water. You can live for forty days without food, but only seven days without water. This is why living water, not just living food, is so important to your Self-Health. One thing you should know is that all water is not created equal. (Water isn't water isn't water.)

Taking Other People's Drugs

Are you taking other people's drugs? If you are drinking your local tap water you are, in all likelihood, drinking other people's drugs. That's not a joke. According to a 2008, five-month investigation by the Associated Press, there is a vast array of pharmaceuticals in our drinking water, including antibiotics, antiseizure medication, mood drugs, mental illness meds, asthma steroids, sex hormones, tranquilizers, heart medicines, and, even more disturbing, chemotherapies and radiation treatments.

The Associated Press researchers tested the water of twenty-four major metropolitan areas and found over 287 different prescribed drugs. Although drugs were found in the water systems of all the cities, some cities had more than others.

It's not just our tap water that is polluted. More than a hundred phar-

maceuticals have been discovered in lakes, rivers, reservoirs, and streams. And the problem isn't confined to surface waters. These drugs have penetrated the nation's deep underground aquifers and springs, the source of 40 percent of the country's drinking water.

Urine Nation of Drugs

Where are all these drugs coming from? Simply put, our urine. When people take drugs, their body absorbs only some of the chemicals; the rest is literally flushed down the toilet. It then goes into the sewer system and out to water treatment plants, which are not equipped to filter drug contaminants before sending the same water back to our homes and faucets. But human waste is not the only source of these drugs; as you know, over half of all pharmaceuticals are fed to the animals of concentration camps and a growing number of pets, who are now being prescribed the same human drugs that their human owners take. This avalanche of drugged-up urine and feces flows into our water systems every single day.

Don't Drink the Water

What do all these drugs do to our bodies? Ask Thomas White, a consultant and spokesman for the pharmaceutical companies. He says, "There's little or no risk from pharmaceuticals in the environment to human health." The pharmaceutical companies claim the concentrations of these drugs are tiny and incapable of causing any harm to animals, humans, or the environment.

Officials at local water utilities also insist that their city's drinking water meets all federal and state regulations, and according to the EPA and FDA, the water is safe for consumption. (Why does that not comfort me?)

Yet while bureaucracies defend their poisons, there is growing concern among many scientists that this poisoned water could cause harm because, unlike most foods, water is consumed in high doses by humans every day. It may be easy for our bodies to shrug off a one-time dose of these drugs, but being exposed to smaller doses on a daily basis over fifty years could indeed be a problem. We also know that ingesting many different drugs at one time can greatly increase their dangerous side effects. The presence of chlorine, which is added to our water by treatment plants, has been found to make many pharmaceuticals even more toxic. For a free full list of the cities tested and the respective drugs found in their drinking water, see our website.

Know Your H$_2$O

Don't drink the poison. The best water to drink is vapor-distilled or reverse-osmosis water, processes that filter out most if not all of the drugs, germs, and poisons found in our water today. Creating healthful water means removing bad things but keeping good things, such as minerals. Water totally stripped of all minerals cannot even sustain the life of the goldfish in your aquarium, much less the human body. Some of the better bottled water companies are restoring important minerals to their filtered water.

There are also some great natural spring–sourced waters, but make sure the bottling location is as remote as possible. The farther the spring is from civilization, the more likely that the water is truly pure. Forty percent of bottled water in our stores today is repackaged tap water. So don't be fooled: be sure to check the labels and the water's source.

Acid (Water) Trip

Another important thing to consider when choosing the right water for your Self-Health is acidity. Much of the water today has become acidic, causing our bodies to gradually become more acidic too. When we are born, we have the highest alkaline mineral concentration and body pH (low acidity) that we will ever have. From our birth forward the growing acidity in our water and foods (due to pollution and toxins) makes us more and more acidic. All this happens without our notice. Consider this: if you drop a frog into a kettle of boiling water, it will immediately jump out. However, if you place the frog in a kettle of lukewarm water and gradually increase the temperature, it will stay in the water until it boils to death.

Many of us are suffering from the effects of long-term, low-grade body acidity. Like the frog, we just don't notice that the water is getting warmer and warmer (more and more acidic). Our lack of energy, aches, pains, indigestion, and mood swings just seem to creep up on us. Our fat cells begin to store the acid that our body cannot dispose of, and we now know that if our body is overly acidic, our cells cannot detoxify properly. Many degenerative diseases may be the result of acid waste buildup within the body. This can lead to weight gain, blood pressure issues, bone loss, kidney wasting, premature aging, and even cancer.

Acidic water holds very little oxygen. Alkaline water can hold large amounts of oxygen. You will find out in the next chapter just how much cancer hates oxygen. In fact, people with cancer tend to have higher blood acidity, lower pH blood levels, and less oxygen in their blood.

Filtered or Bottled Is Best

If you cannot afford to purchase bottled water, you can pick up a home filtration system. Prices vary, and though these faucet systems may set you back a few bucks, they are worth the expense. I have a filtration system at home and drink a good bit of healthful bottled water as well. My favorite water is Essentia because it has a very high pH level (meaning it is nonacidic) and powerful antioxidant qualities and is full of electrolytes, which allow us to absorb more water quickly into our system. Essentia can be found at your local health food store or grocery. You can get more information on our website.

You should also focus on eating water-rich foods like lettuce, watermelon, oranges, apples, grapefruits, cantaloupe, carrots, broccoli, cherries, blueberries, and strawberries. These foods are 70 percent water and include lots of minerals and plant chemicals. For a free list of the best filtered water

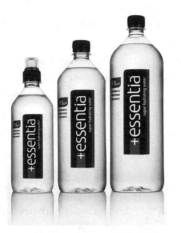

and a side-by-side bottled water comparison chart, please visit our website.

Do You Have a Drinking Problem?

Do you drink too much (or too little)? Most people think they drink enough water, but they don't. I used to think that unless my mouth was dry I didn't need to drink anything. Sound familiar? Dry mouth is not the only way your body tells you that you are thirsty. In fact, the older you get, the less likely you are to know when you are dehydrated. And when your body does tell you that you need water, it may actually speak to you through pain rather than dry mouth.

When there is a shortage of water in the body, some parts are forced to go without because the brain will ration water to the most important parts first. In a freezing snowstorm, the first body parts to lose heat are the fingers and limbs because the brain can survive without them. In the same way, those lower priority areas of the body suffering from drought are faced with dehydration, and the way the body lets you know about it is with localized pain.

Many people who suffer from chronic pains such as headaches are simply dehydrated. Improving water intake has been found to help with heartburn, arthritis, back pain, chest pain, stomach pains, asthma, high blood pressure, diabetes, and high cholesterol. Remember, one of the two primary causes of disease is poison (toxins). Your body needs water to flush those poisons out of your system. When poisons are not removed from the body, inflammation and pain will result. If you're experiencing pain, your body may simply be crying out for you to drink more water.

The River of Life

Did you know that there is a mysterious river (twice as large as your blood system) flowing throughout your body? This river picks up all the pollutants (poisons, toxins, waste, viruses, bacteria) in the body at over six hundred different sites (the lymph nodes) and dumps them into a drain (the thoracic duct) located next to the heart; it is about the size of your pinkie. This river of life is the heart and soul of your

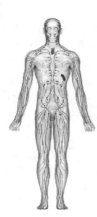

immune system. It sweeps out toxins, filters out infections, takes poisons to the liver for cleansing and to the kidneys for elimination. It basically takes out our garbage.

This lymph river snakes through our bodies and through hundreds of mesh-like tissues called nodes. These nodes are loaded with killer cells that catch and kill germs and toxins. You may have noticed some of these nodes, such as the ones under the back of your jawbone or along your neck that swell when you are sick.

Unlike the blood system, which is powered by the heart, this river of life has no pump to create flow. It relies mainly on our body's movement and our water intake to keep its flow of garbage moving. Just like a river during a drought, if we are dehydrated the flow weakens and garbage accumulates rather than being washed downstream and out of the body. Where this garbage settles, inflammation occurs,

which, over time, can turn into disease, even cancer.

The body also uses water to produce energy. All of our body's electrical energy from its 4 trillion nerve and brain cells comes from water power (hydrolysis). So if you are weak and tired before the end of the work day, or stressed, anxious, or depressed, or you find yourself craving caffeine, alcohol, or even drugs, it could simply be your body begging you for water.

Don't Wait to Get Thirsty

How much water should you drink? You should drink about half your weight in ounces every day. So if you weigh 100 pounds, you should be drinking 50 ounces of water a day. I know that may sound like a lot, but it's truly what your body needs. Try it for ten days and see what happens. You should drink some water every two hours because it takes about that long to use up (evaporate) the water you drank two hours earlier. (You need more water if it's hot or if you're exercising.) You should drink water as soon as you wake up, since your body has gone several hours without it. You should also drink water before and after eating because your body uses water to break down food into nutrients. The body also uses water to break down fats. Many people who increase their daily water intake will automatically lose weight as well.

What Color Is Your Urine?

How do you know if you're getting enough water? Look at your urine. If it's clear in color, then you are probably getting enough (unless you are drinking a lot of caffeine, which will also make your urine clear). If your urine is yellow, then you are moderately dehydrated. If it's orange or darker, then you are extremely dehydrated.

Drink Half Your Weight in Water for Ten Days

Whatever the color of your urine, get living water into your body. Get yourself some bottled water or filter your own water at home and fill your bottles to take to work with you or wherever you go. You will soon have more energy, lose weight, push out pollutants, rid yourself of pain, and ward off disease. Make sure you get your water from the right source. Don't be fooled. Protect your Self-Health.

So for the next ten days, drink enough water to equal half your weight in ounces. Divide your weight by 2, and drink that number in ounces.

Drain Your Lymph Lake

Due to lack of water and body movement, our lymph river sometimes resembles a stagnant lake or swamp. Giving your body external pressure and joint movement is often needed to kick-start its crucial flow. Massage and chiropractic manipulation can be extraordinary tools to help drain your lymph lake and get your river flowing. They both improve nervous, circulatory, and lymphatic system flow and truly awaken the healer within. If you have not been to a masseuse or chiropractor in a while, or ever, this might be a good time to plan a visit.

Living Oxygen

The human body can live for forty days without food, seven days without water, but only five minutes without oxygen. Oxygen is the one thing our body needs the most, yet it is something we often take for granted. I breathe in, I breathe out. What's there to think about? Our lungs are pretty much on autopilot. There is nothing for us to do. Or is there?

The lungs have no muscle of their own; they are like two loose, empty sacks. The movement of the diaphragm, the large muscle within the rib cage, is what draws air in and out of the lungs, much like a bellows. The diaphragm moves automatically, without our having to think about it. A more controlled, conscious effort can make the diaphragm draw oxygen much farther into the lower lungs, pushing it much more deeply into the cells.

Take a Big Hit of O$_2$

A person taking a hit of marijuana breathes in deeply, expanding his diaphragm, and holds his breath for a long time so that the smoke will go deep into his lungs and thus into his cells. Using the same method, you can greatly increase the amount of oxygen that your body absorbs by consciously using your diaphragm to take in more air.

The richest blood flow is in the lower lungs, so if we fail to get air into this area, we will not get the maximum amount of oxygen into our body. Many of us are missing 20 to 30 percent of the oxygen we should be getting to our cells because we never use our diaphragm to breathe deeply. The average person reaches peak lung function and capacity in his mid-twenties and then loses up to 25 percent lung capacity every ten years thereafter.

Shallow breathing limits the amount of oxygen in your blood, so toxins build up in your cells. Your lungs are one of the primary ways your body gets rid of waste, and if they are not exhaling fully, you feel sluggish, weak, tired. Over time, your organs begin to suffer, your cells get less and less oxygen, your heart is overworked, your brain—which is only 2 percent of total body weight but consumes 25 percent of the body's oxygen—becomes sluggish, and you store fat instead of burning it, causing weight gain.

Cancer Hates Oxygen

This explains why many people are living an *anaerobic* lifestyle, which means they are not taking in enough oxygen. Their breathing is shallow, and they spend hours, days, weeks, perhaps even months without deep, healthful breathing. This means that oxygen never penetrates their lower lungs, never reaches the richest blood supply, and so their cells lack precious oxygen. We know that all normal cells require oxygen, but did you know that cancer cells can only live without oxygen?

Tests have shown that if you deprive a normal human cell of 35 percent of its oxygen, it will become cancerous within forty-eight hours; deprive a cell of 60 percent of its oxygen, and it will become cancerous in a matter of hours. When the oxygen saturation of blood falls because of constant shallow breathing, conditions in cells become ripe for cancer.

Our bodies were designed for deep breathing. Remember our hunter-gatherer ancestors? They experienced deep breathing daily if not hourly as they worked with their hands, toiled in their organic gardens, and chased down wild game. For most of us, our lifestyles are designed for shallow breathing. Our moments of deepest breathing come when we get up from our desks and computer screens to fetch a cup of coffee, yell at a coworker or family member who has upset us, or frantically run the trash out of the house just in time to catch the garbage truck.

As I sit here in front of my own computer, I know how hard it can be to escape the shallow breathing lifestyle. But what happens if we don't find a way to break free of our cubicles and start breathing deeply again, the way we were created to do?

Breathe Deeply

All you need is fifteen minutes a day to start an aerobic (meaning "with oxygen") deep-breathing lifestyle. That's right. Take fifteen minutes out of your day and go for a short walk—before work, during lunch, after work, following dinner, whenever, wherever. Get out of your cubicle, office, living room, closet, or cave and get out into the sun-

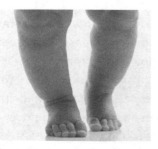

light. See and enjoy the fresh air, birds, flowers, sights and sounds, and walk—and breathe deeply.

If it helps, start off walking slowly, and as you get fitter, walk faster; you may eventually want to start jogging or even running. You might like it so much you'll extend your exercise for thirty minutes or longer. The important thing is to start to breathe deeply now. Determine when you are going to do it, and commit to a fifteen-minute walk every day for ten days.

If you do, within a few days you will notice that you have more energy, more enthusiasm, and more stamina; your muscles will become toned, you will begin to get thinner, and you will sleep much better. You will lower your risk of stroke, heart attack, high blood pressure, diabetes, and cancer. More than 30 percent of people in America today get cancer. Athletes who breathe deeply when they exercise every day push their cancer risk down to an incredible 12 percent. Because their built-in bellows (the diaphragm) are pumping massive amounts of oxygen into their lower lungs, they have as much as 25 percent more oxygen in their blood than their shallow-breathing nonathlete counterparts. In just a few weeks you could join their ranks and their statistics. Start today! Try it for ten days and see how you feel.

Yoga: The Art of Breathing

I know what you may be thinking: There he goes, off into Eastern philosophy. (Next he'll be chanting.) Give me a chance to explain. Yoga, often misunderstood by those who have not practiced it, is perhaps one of the best exercises for getting the most amount of oxygen into your lungs. We use only about 20 percent of our lungs' capacity to breathe. Learning how to breathe properly and expand our lungs fully is the heart and soul of the practice of yoga. Classes generally last from thirty minutes to an hour, are fairly inexpensive, and offer a great workout. Sign up and go for a session, learn the art of breathing, and don't worry about becoming a monk or yogi. Just go for the oxygen.

Age Without Aging

Most of us would like to live as long as we can, feeling as young as we can. We would like to be in great health until we are a hundred years old and then die peacefully of old age—just go to sleep and not wake up. That's not such an impossible dream. It could be a reality if we commit ourselves to our own Self-Health.

In his incredible book *UltraPrevention,* Dr. Mark Hyman relates a story of the Tarahumara Indians of Mexico. These Indians are runners. They don't ride horses or mules; they run everywhere they go, long distances from one remote village to another. They have been known to run over sixty miles nonstop in one single hunt. Over the centuries they have truly become the perfect runners. In this village of super-runners, guess who are the best? Believe it or not, it's the old men. In fact, a team of Harvard researchers confirmed this by traveling to Mexico and testing the physiological strength (breathing, fitness, heart, etc.) of the Tarahumara. Astonishingly, the sixty-year-olds were in better shape than the forty-year-olds, who were in better shape than the twenty-year-olds.

A biographer of Alexander the Great tells us that a large percentage of Alexander's Macedonian soldiers were over sixty and could march thirty miles in the desert with a full pack. This group of olive oil– and grape-loving men was the army that conquered the world. Don't tell these men that weakness from aging is inevitable.

Eat Like a Bird, Age Like a Tortoise

Of all of the things you can start doing right now to increase your life span and slow down the aging process, by far the most powerful is simply to eat less food, especially fake food. The average person will consume over seventy tons of food in a lifetime. An excessive amount of food is the single greatest drain on your body. The more you eat, the more your body has to work and expend its life force. Study after study has shown that if you eat 30 percent less food than you do right now, you can extend your life up to 30 percent. It's that simple. Eat less—live longer! The less energy your body has to use to digest food over the years, the more energy it will have for fighting disease and aging. Okinawans, the longest living, healthiest people on the planet, have a saying, *Hara harchi bu,* which means "Eat only until you are 80 percent full." There must be something to it, as their average life span is nearly a hundred years.

For most people, the idea of eating less is not easily digested. (Pardon the pun.) But it's not as hard as you might think. First off, if you're on the Self-Health diet, you are already eating lots of living fruits and vegetables, which are virtually impossible to OD on. You can have an all-you-can-eat buffet on these healthful goodies every single day. You can have your fill and not gain

a pound or drain your life force because they are full of enzymes and easily digested.

You can also learn to eat more slowly. It takes twenty minutes for your brain to recognize that your stomach is full, so give it time to catch up with your eating. If you eat your entire meal in ten minutes, it's too late to stop eating.

Americans tend to eat until the food on their plate runs out. We were taught from our youth to clean our plates. We were never told to stop eating when we feel full. Learn to listen to your belly and brain; they will tell you when you're full, and when they do, stop eating. If you focus more on the quality of your food (organics, wild-caught, locally produced, etc.), you may have less food on your plate, but this food is so much more nutrient-dense that your body will no longer crave massive portions. (And you will possess a superpower over all-you-can-eat buffets.)

You might be thinking, *I don't want*

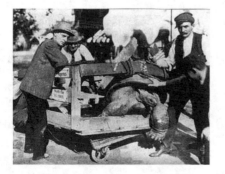

Giant Tortoise, 300 years old, the oldest living animal. Weighing 1,700 pounds and measuring seven feet across the shell, this enormous beast broke the box trying to get out at the 1904 St. Louis World's Fair.

to eat like a bird. Believe it or not, birds actually consume about half their body weight in food each day. They go bananas for living foods and fresh water and get tons of aerobic exercise by flapping their wings. So eat like a bird (go crazy on water, fruits, and veggies), and you will age like a tortoise.

They live up to three hundred years on fruits and veggies.

Yet even if you eat like a bird, get plenty of oxygen into your lungs, and drink the purest water in the world, it still may not be enough to save your Self-Health. In the next chapter I will tell you why.

Self-Health Summary: The Ten-Day Challenge

5 Things Your Body Must Have Every Day (from chapter 10)

FEVPO =   **F**ruits (Eat widely)
Enzymes (Broad spectrum)
Vegetables (Eat widely)
Probiotics (Broad spectrum)
Oils (Pristine source)

2 Things You Must Do Every Day to Get FEVPO (from chapter 10)

• 15 Minute Self-Health Smoothie (recipe in chapter 15)
• 15 Minute Self-Health Salad (recipe in chapter 15)

Next Self-Health Steps

• Living H_2O (drink half your weight in ounces of alkaline water)
• Living O_2 (start with fifteen minutes of walking and deep breathing every day)

CHAPTER TWELVE

Guard Your Heart

Above all else, guard your heart for it is the wellspring of life.
—King Solomon

Ultimately the most important thing I can tell you about Self-Health has nothing to do with what you put in your mouth but what you have in your heart. You can eat the greatest living foods gathered from the four corners of the Earth, but if your heart is not right, you will not find Self-Health.

Your heart is the source of your deepest emotions, feelings, character, and beliefs. Often overlooked, the heart is important above all else. This fact simply cannot be overstated or exaggerated. To protect your Self-Health, you must also protect your heart from the spiritual poisons that can make it sick, and that can make your body sick as well. Poisons like stress, worry, anger, resentment, negativity, and depression can damage you and hinder progress in your mental and physical health. So Self-Health is not just about what you are eating; it's also about what's eating you.

Cigarettes and Happiness

Which do you think can lower your life expectancy more: smoking or unhappiness? Would you believe they both harm you equally? They both shorten your life by roughly ten years. According to recent studies, smoking two packs of cigarettes a day has the same effect on how long you will live as having a negative view on life. Wow! That's powerful. If that's the case, we should

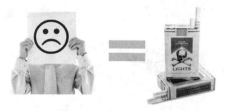

demand public awareness campaigns on human unhappiness as well as antismoking ads.

Drugging Our Depression

A survey released by the American Psychological Association reveals that one-third of all people today are extremely stressed (23 percent of women and 19 percent of men feel super-stressed). Twenty million people now suffer from some form of depression, and the rate of depression among children is an astounding 23 percent.

The most widely prescribed drugs in America today are antidepressants: 118 million prescriptions annually. According to the Centers for Disease Control, antidepressive drugs are prescribed more than medications for high blood pressure, cholesterol, asthma, ulcers, sexual dysfunction, or even headaches.

And here's a shock: preschoolers are the fastest-growing market for antidepressants. At least 4 percent of preschoolers—over a million kids—are clinically depressed and on drugs. Yet studies have shown most antidepressants are no more effective in curing depression than sugar pills (placebos). They do, however, make pharmaceutical companies a great deal of money.

The Health of Happiness

Does unhappiness actually affect our health? According to the American Psychological Association, 43 percent of adults suffer adverse health effects from stress, 33 percent of all doctor visits are for stress-related causes, and all six of the leading causes of death (heart disease, cancer, lung ailments, liver disease, accidents, and suicide) have been linked to or are induced by stress. By 2020 (at its current pace) depression will be the second largest killer after heart disease. Americans are literally dying from unhappiness.

Poisons of the heart (unhappiness, stress, worry, anger, resentment, negativity) all cause dis-ease in our body,

To avoid sickness, eat less; to prolong life, worry less.
—CHU HUI WENG,
CHINESE PHILOSOPHER

lowering our immune system, raising our adrenaline levels, and ultimately creating a toxic environment under our skin. It is a scientific fact that people who are happy get sick less often, recover faster, accomplish more, and live much longer. Happiness of the heart by any measure is necessary for Self-Health.

Hunting Happiness

Are you happy? Honestly? Despite the fact that we have a constitutional right to pursue happiness, few Americans actually think they have found it. Happiness for many of us has proven to be elusive, momentary, and fleeting at best. Many of us believe happiness will come when we accomplish a certain dream or goal or acquire some desired object. We work, strive, achieve, stress, and worry until we get what we are after (or die trying). What happens when we get what we want? What comes next? Happiness? Martin Seligman, a psychologist and professor, recounts what happens in one such story in his powerful book, *Authentic Happiness:*

> Ruth, a single mother in the Hyde Park neighborhood of Chicago, needed more hope in her life, and she got it cheaply by buying five dollars' worth of lottery tickets every week. She needed large doses of hope because her usual mood was low (and had been) . . . at least since middle school twenty years ago. . . . Then a miracle happened: Ruth won 22 million dollars in the Illinois state lottery. She was beside herself with joy. She quit her gift-wrapping job at Neiman-Marcus, and bought an eighteen-room house in Evanston, a Versace wardrobe, and a robin's-egg-blue Jaguar. She was even able to send her twin sons to a private school. Strangely, however, as the year went by, her mood drifted downward. By the end of the year, in spite of the absence of any obvious adversity, her expensive therapist diagnosed her as having depression.

She had everything she wanted but was still unhappy. How could this be?

Chasing Mirages

A recent study of twenty-two people who had won large amounts of money in major lotteries found that within a relatively short period of time, all twenty-two reverted to their previous level of happiness, winding up no happier than they were before. Should this surprise us? Think about your own life. Have you ever received something that you really wanted? How did it make you feel? At first it feels great, truly wonderful. And then what? After a while,

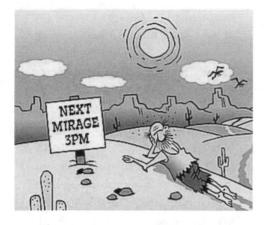

I saw a man pursuing the horizon;
Round and round they sped.
I was disturbed at this;
I accosted the man.
"It is futile," I said,
"You can never—"

"You lie," he cried,
And ran on.

you begin to take it for granted. As we get more and more stuff and do more and more things, our expectations rise. We need something even bigger to satisfy us and boost our level of happiness back up to where it was before. Once we acquire our next possession or reach a higher-level achievement, we get used to that too, and quickly look for our next "happiness fix."

This happiness roller coaster is never-ending. It's not unlike a drug. When it wears off, you need another bump. Pursuing happiness can be like chasing a mirage in the desert. Upon arriving at the imagined oasis, we realize it's not what we had thought. Then we see another beautiful oasis in the distance, and with little thought we start running toward the next mirage. Many people spend their whole lives chasing such mirages in search of happiness. They are like the man in Stephen Crane's poem:

Studies clearly show that people who have more good things in life are no happier than the less fortunate. In less than three months most new events, no matter how positive, begin to lose their impact. Good things and incredible accomplishments have little power to raise the level of happiness in our hearts for more than a short while. Wealth does not bring happiness. Income has grown dramatically in this country in the past fifty years, but our happiness level has not kept pace.

Other factors, such as physical attractiveness, fame, talent, and power, do not have much of a long-term effect on happiness either. The people who have these things know this to be true. They have arrived at perhaps the ultimate mirage and realize that it's not what they had imagined. Deep down we all know this to be true. There are people who seemingly have it all—the best job, great looks, a perfect spouse, lots of friends, power, and prestige—but one day their life crumbles. Something happens, perhaps a divorce, drug use, depression, or even suicide, revealing that this person was actually extremely unhappy. Are we that different? Remember that time when you finally got what you wanted? How many days, weeks, or months did it make you happy? How long did it take for you to seek something new? What makes us think the next thing will satisfy any more than the last?

Does Your Past Predict Your Future?

Happiness of the heart that leads to Self-Health is not found in possessions, accomplishments, or any external circumstance. Health of the heart is something that happens from the inside out. Happiness is determined by how we handle our circumstances rather than by the circumstances themselves. We all carry around some baggage from our past: broken homes, abusive relationships, disappointments, failures, hurts, guilt, fears. Many people believe that their past predicts their future. Do you?

Charles Darwin taught us many years ago that we are the sum of our past victories. The strongest will always survive and win because they always have. (The past predicts the future.) That doesn't give much hope to those of us who have had less than a perfect past, does it? Then Sigmund Freud came along and told us that every future psychological event in our lives is determined by what happened in our past. Again, we are being told that our past determines our future. Freud's powerful influence, even today, has many people spending their lives attempting to fix some unresolved childhood trauma in order to find and fulfill their happiness as an adult.

The Real Freudian Slip

With all due respect to Freud (and Freudians), the truth is, as recent studies have shown, our childhood traumas have little determining influence on our adult happiness. This is not hard to believe. We all know people who had a horrible childhood but were deter-

> *Happiness cannot be traveled to, owned, earned, worn or consumed. Happiness is the spiritual experience of living every minute with love, grace and gratitude.*
> —DENIS WAITLEY,
> MOTIVATOR AND AUTHOR

mined to become happy, healthy, positive, and productive people despite their upbringing. They became successful at being happy and positive without blaming their parents, abuse, stress, spouse, sex, drugs, alcohol, hurts, failures, injustice, or childhood. Perhaps you are one of those self-driven, happy people.

All too often in life we can become bitter about our past and hopeless about our future, believing those negative events in our personal history have somehow imprisoned us and doomed us to failure, or at least to mediocrity. We allow our joy, contentment, and happiness to be stolen by thoughts that emphasize the bad things in our lives without fully appreciating the good things.

Are You Talking (to Yourself) Too Much?

Do you talk to yourself? Everybody does. In fact, research shows the average person talks to himself 50,000 times a day. And guess what? Eighty percent of what we say to ourselves is negative. We tell ourselves things like *Everyone always takes advantage of me. I never get any time for myself. They don't like me. That was a dumb thing to say. This outfit doesn't look good on me. I'll never be a good dancer. No one ever notices me. Nobody cares if I live or die. I bet I look fat. I'll never lose this weight.*

There's no way I can do this Self-Health thing. I'll never change. And on and on it goes. No wonder we're not happy.

Many of us constantly bombard ourselves with negative thoughts and beliefs. If someone else said these things to us, we would become angry, but because the indictment comes from our own heart, we believe the attacks to be true. Things we say to ourselves are rarely challenged. Most people are not even consciously aware that their inner voice is speaking to them, much less aware of what it might be saying. It is so innate and automatic that whatever it says immediately becomes unquestioned reality. Do you know what you say to yourself? Can you hear your own voice? Is it telling you the truth?

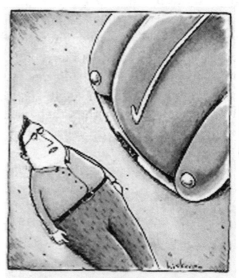

Encumbered by a low self-image, Bob takes a job as a speed bump.

www.Qigmans.com

The problem with believing everything you say to yourself is that sometimes your inner voice can be wrong. Beliefs are just that: beliefs. They may or may not be true. Can you think of a time when your inner voice was wrong? It told you one thing, you believed it, and then you found out that the opposite was true? Just because a person's inner voice tells him he is unlovable, unemployable, unforgivable, or inadequate doesn't mean that it's true. This judgmental voice that we allow to have free rein in our heads is not infallible and must be challenged. We need to learn to argue with this constantly critical voice.

The Art of Debating Yourself

The most convincing way to argue with your inner voice is to prove it to be factually incorrect. Play the role of a defense attorney and ask, "What is the evidence for this belief?" If you think your grade on a test was the worst in the class, check the evidence. Did the person next to you get a lower grade? If you believe you blew your Self-Health diet by eating some chicken wings, compare that one little infraction with how much bet-

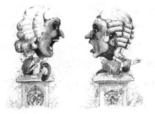

ter you have been eating this week. The point is, don't give your critical inner voice a free ride. Make it prove itself.

Look for alternative interpretations of a potentially negative event. We tend to latch on to the worst belief possible, not because of evidence but precisely because it's the most catastrophic belief and the one we fear the most. Ask yourself, "Are there any alternatives to this negative belief?" If your inner voice says, "You're the worst student in the class," then ask yourself if this exam was especially difficult. Perhaps you didn't know you would have to prepare that much, or maybe the teacher graded you unfairly. It's very possible that the first interpretation that comes to your mind after an event is probably the most negative one and not to be trusted.

Sometimes when you argue with yourself, the facts are not on your side.

Don't believe everything you hear . . . even in your mind.
—DANIEL G. AMEN, MD

You checked the facts, and your inner voice is right. That's when you calmly ask yourself, "What are the implications?" One bad grade does not mean you are a bad student. One chicken wing does not mean you are a failure at Self-Health. Again, the tendency of our inner voice, even if it's right about the facts, is to exaggerate the implications and jump immediately to the worst-case scenario. You should ask yourself, "How likely is the worst case to happen?" According to the facts, what are the more likely scenarios? Tell yourself, *FEAR stands for fantasized experiences appearing real*. Don't let your inner voice doom you to fear and failure.

Stomp on Your ANTs

Dr. Daniel G. Amen, a psychiatrist, calls these limiting inner thoughts ANTs (automatic negative thoughts), and just like ants at a picnic (or in your pants), these ANTs can ruin your day and your life. Dr. Amen says we should learn to deal with our ANTs by becoming aware that they exist, shaking them off, squashing them by challenging them, and then replacing them with more positive and affirming thoughts. We must realize we are in control of our thoughts. Whether or not we will listen to or agree with our inner voice is clearly within our power. Ask yourself, *Is this belief hurting or helping me? Is it getting me closer to what I want, or farther away? Is it empowering me to take action or freezing me with fear and self-doubt?*

Over the next ten days, argue with your ANTs. Get a notebook and write down all the ANTs that come to your mind, and then practice disputing them. Talk back to your ANTs, challenge their truth, question their reality, consider more positive alternative interpretations, and stomp on unfounded attacks that are hostile to your goals and dreams.

Want to know more about how to stomp your ANTs successfully and make your self-talk more positive? Check out our free tools online.

> *A man is literally what he thinks. You are today where your thoughts have brought you; you will be tomorrow where your thoughts take you.*
>
> —JAMES ALLEN,
> AUTHOR OF *AS A MAN THINKETH*

CHAPTER THIRTEEN

THE SECRET TO HAPPINESS:
Gratitude and Forgiveness

A merry heart does good like a medicine:
but a broken spirit dries up the bones.
—King Solomon

The two culprits that steal our joy, contentment, and happiness are an overemphasis on bad things in our lives and an underappreciation of the good things. The two antidotes to these poisons of the heart, as ancient and simple as they may sound, are gratitude and forgiveness. Gratitude amplifies your appreciation of the good things in your life (past and present), and forgiveness lessens the power of the bad things to make you bitter and can even change those hurtful memories into good ones.

Forgiveness = Health?

You might be wondering, *What's forgiveness doing in a Self-Health book?*

Would you believe me if I told you that forgiveness can improve cardiovascular function, diminish chronic pain, relieve depression, and boost the quality of life among the very ill? It's true.

Everett Worthington Jr., a professor at Virginia Commonwealth University and the author of *Five Steps to Forgiveness: The Art and Science of Forgiving,* is also a clinical psychologist and a pioneer in forgiveness research. He has found that people who don't forgive have more stress-related disorders, lower immune system function, and a higher rate of cardiovascular disease and other illnesses. Those who have found a way to pardon the transgressions of others experience lower blood pressure, less depression, and better overall mental and physical health than those who do not forgive easily.

Science is now proving that forgiving others is no longer solely a balm for the soul but is also, and more powerfully, medicine for the body. Just like eating living foods, drinking enough water, breathing deeply, and exercising, forgiveness appears to be a behavior that a person can learn, practice, and repeat as needed to prevent disease and preserve Self-Health.

Does it surprise you to learn that forgiveness has such a powerful effect on our health and happiness? So many people carry around the pain, abuse, hurts, disappointments, and resentments of the past. It is evident in their face, their body, their personality, and their words. These people will never be free to be healthy or happy in the present or the future as long as they are anchored in the past.

Why We Don't Forgive

Whether or not you agree that forgiveness is necessary for your Self-Health, you can surely agree that forgiving is difficult business. Why is it so hard for us to forgive? Many times we don't just hold on to bitterness, we passionately embrace it. If forgiveness is so healing for our heart and healthful for our body, why does forgiveness not come more naturally?

Unfortunately our inner voice gives us what might seem to be very good reasons to hold on to our hurts. For example, forgiving is truly unjust. Justice demands wrongdoers should pay for their sins. Forgiveness seems to negate justice and contradicts the righteous indignation we feel when we are offended or see others mistreated. When we forgive, we sometimes feel we are being disloyal to the victim (even if we ourselves are the victim).

Perhaps the hardest part about forgiving is that it makes us feel vulnerable to being hurt or disappointed yet again. You know the old saying: Fool me once, shame on you; fool me twice, shame on me. Yet it is possible for us to forgive someone 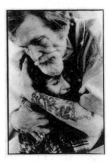 without putting ourselves into a situation where he can hurt us in the same way again.

Forgiving is not about saving the person who inflicted the pain. It's really about saving ourselves. We can't hurt the person who hurt us by not forgiving, but we can set ourselves free from a dark and bitter future by choosing to forgive him. When we swallow the poison pill of unforgiveness, it poisons us, not the other person. When we truly understand this, we realize that we have no choice but to forgive, for not

> *Resentment is like drinking poison and then hoping it will kill your enemies.*
>
> —NELSON MANDELA

doing so would be a form of emotional suicide.

Five Steps to Save Yourself with Forgiveness

In his book *Five Steps to Forgiveness*, Everett Worthington describes a five-step process to forgiveness he calls REACH. He knows about the subject. On New Year's morning in 1996, he found his aged mother brutally beaten to death with a crowbar and a baseball bat. In the attack, she had been raped with a wine bottle. REACH came from his own successful struggle to forgive the criminals who killed his beloved mother.

R stands for *Recall the hurt*. Try to think about your hurt as objectively as you can without emotion. Do not allow yourself to become angry, to think of the other person as evil, or to sink in the mire of self-pity.

E stands for *Empathize with the person who hurt you*. Ask yourself, Why did this person hurt me? What was going on in his life that might have caused him to do such a thing? Hurt people

hurt people: people strike out when they are scared, worried, and in pain. All people are capable of doing unbelievable things when they fear for their own survival. Unless we have walked in another's shoes, it's hard to know what has made him the way he is. Think about how people sometimes define you in a way that gives no thought to where you have come from or what you have been through. Keep in mind that people sometimes hurt others deeply without even being aware of the pain they have caused.

A stands for *Give the altruistic (selfless) gift of forgiveness*. This is a hard one. Try to think of a time that you did something really wrong to someone, and he forgave you. Do you remember how guilty you felt? Do you recall how much you wanted and needed his forgiveness? He gave you something you did not deserve. You received a gift that he did not have to give. Is it right to refuse to share a gift that was freely given to you? If you hurt someone in the future (and you will), how can you ever hope for or ask for his forgiveness if you are not willing to give it yourself? These are hard questions, but we must ask them if we are to free ourselves from the pain of the past and embrace an incredible future of happiness and Self-Health.

C stands for *Commit yourself to forgive publicly*. Worthington tells his listeners to write "a certificate of forgiveness," which is a letter, poem, or song written directly to the offender, or in your personal diary, or read to a close friend.

H stands for *Hold onto forgiveness*. Old memories of the hurts of the past will raise their ugly heads in the future. We can forgive, but it's hard to forget. Forgiveness can't erase the pictures that pop into your head, but it can change the captions written on them. Memories don't mean you have not forgiven, so don't wallow in them. Release those thoughts, and remember, you have already forgiven.

For more free info on forgiveness, go to our website.

No Motivational Gobbledygook

I realize that, for some of you, this information on forgiveness may seem a little mushy or touchy-feely. I can certainly understand your feeling that way, but just like everything I have challenged you to do for your Self-Health, I urge you to put it to the test. This is not some motivational gobbledygook where you recite positive statements like "Every day, in every way, I'm getting better and better." This is about real, hard, gut-wrenching change. This is about healing your heart and soul, and thus your body.

Over the next ten days I dare you to forgive. Go through the steps to REACH. Write that letter of forgiveness to someone who has wronged you. See how it makes you feel. What if it truly frees you from past resentments and hurts? What if it fills you with a sense of peace and contentment? Thousands of people have experienced amazing physical changes (weight loss, lower blood pressure, decreased chronic illness, reduced heart problems, cancer in remission) within days or weeks of simply forgiving. Prove me wrong! Try giving the gift of forgiveness for the next ten days. If you do, you will find that it's actually a gift that you give to yourself.

> *He who refuses to forgive, burns the bridge over which he too must one day cross.*
>
> —AUTHOR UNKNOWN

> *If the only prayer you said in your whole life was "Thank you," that would suffice.*
>
> —MEISTER ECKHART,
> GERMAN THEOLOGIAN AND PHILOSOPHER

Gratitude: The Granddaddy of Happiness

Do you need a "gratitude adjustment"? I realize this may sound a little corny. I know it may seem a lot more fun to be cynical. It's easy to emphasize the negative and ignore the positive. That's what most people do, but then again, most people aren't very happy. Gratitude teaches us to focus on the good things in our life and is absolutely necessary for our Self-Health. Why do you think all the psychologists, philosophers, and religious teachers from Buddha to Jesus to Gandhi have elevated gratitude as one of the highest virtues of all, and the one most closely associated with true happiness? In 43 BC Cicero, the greatest orator in Rome, wrote, "Gratitude is not only the greatest of virtues, but the parent of all the others."

The Grace of Gratitude

Gratitude comes from the Latin word *gratia*, which simply means "grace." It means you are constantly aware of the good things in your life and you don't take them for granted. Gratitude possesses a sense of wonder, awe, appreciation, and thankfulness for life itself. It is the quality that enables you to stop and smell the roses, enjoying and noticing the everyday things. It's feeling a real sense of appreciation for the people in your life and an ever-present understanding of what your life would be without them. Gratitude knows deep inside that life is an undeserved gift that God has given you and you're lucky to be alive at this time in history, living where you are, doing what you're doing, being with the people you are with. It's the realization that your life is so much more blessed than that of

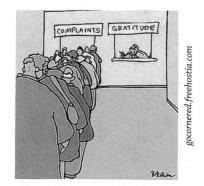

gocornered.freehostia.com

billions of others who have walked this earth.

Gratitude is not directed at yourself but at everything outside of you that you are privileged to experience. It's the absence of self-awareness, self-focus, and self-obsession. It is impossible to know gratitude and self-obsession at the same time; they cannot occupy the same space simultaneously.

No Psycho Mumbo Jumbo

This may all sound too deep, like some kind of psycho mumbo jumbo, but think about it—it's really just common sense and something all of us have already experienced and know in our hearts to be true. Think of a time in your life when you were truly grateful. Maybe you came close to death, or you almost lost someone dear to you, or perhaps something so wonderful happened to you that it humbled you and made you realize you were undeserving. We all have these moments. And that's just it—they are only moments. Like a beautiful butterfly that softly alights on our hands just for a moment, then suddenly flutters off on the breeze. It leaves as quickly as it came, and its beauty is soon forgotten. Many of us go through huge swaths of experience on automatic pilot, without thinking, noticing, or appreciating the richness of our lives.

Practice, Practice, Practice

How do we seize the moment, get off this maddening treadmill, and enjoy the peace, happiness, and contentment (Self-Health) that gratitude undeniably brings? Practice is the answer. Practice being grateful every day. Imagine: What if you did not have the things you now have? What about the people in your life? What if you lost your job, your house, your family, your spouse, your best friend? What would life be like? What if you went home and no one was there, there was no one to talk to or to share your life with?

We usually experience these feelings only when we actually lose something of value. Then it's too late to show our appreciation. I remember how I felt when my father died. I had no idea how much he really meant to me until he was gone. I was standing on his shoulders without even realizing it, until he was tragically pulled out from under me. So do it now. Don't wait for death or some other catastrophe to jolt you off autopilot.

It's interesting that in our culture we do not have a tradition or vehicle for telling people how thankful we are for them and how much they truly mean to us while they are still alive. In fact, when we are moved emotionally and it involuntarily comes out, everyone involved is embarrassed and quickly tries to put the moment behind them. How many times have you been at a funeral and thought, *I wish he was alive to hear this. If only he could know how appreciated he was.* Instead of waiting for the funeral, why not practice now how you would feel if you lost him.

Have a "Gratitude Night"

The psychologist Martin Seligman asked his students to select an important person in their life, present or past, who had made a positive difference to them and to whom the student had never fully expressed thanks. He asked them to write a one-page letter to this person. When he told the students to take their time working on the assignment, most of them took several weeks. When the letters were finished, he told them to laminate the letter and present it as a gift to the person. Seligman stressed that it was important to do so face to face and not in writing or over the phone. The students were not to tell the person the purpose of their visit in advance—a simple "I just want to see you" would work fine. "When all has settled down," Seligman instructed, "read your letter out loud slowly, with expression and eye contact. Then let the other person respond unhurriedly. Reminisce together about the events that make this person so important to you."

After everyone in the class had completed the process, Seligman asked them all to gather for what they would forever remember as "Gratitude Night." The impact was dramatic. As students recounted the stories that inspired their gratitude letters, there was not a dry eye in the classroom, including Seligman's. Something had happened to these students in the simple act of writing these letters that had touched the great emotional underpinnings of life itself: they had experienced gratitude. At the year-end evaluations, it was not uncommon for students to write, "Friday, October 27th (Gratitude Night), was the greatest day of my life."

We don't have to go back to college or join Dr. Seligman's classroom to benefit from the lessons learned from this amazing experiment. Why not write your own gratitude letter? Think of someone important to you, and write him a letter. Let him know how you feel while he is still alive. Decide to start now. If you put it off, it will never get done. Just start writing the letter now and you can decide later how and when to talk with this person.

Start a Gratitude Journal

Another way Seligman suggests we can experience appreciation and gratitude is to set aside five minutes each night for the next ten days and think back over the previous twenty-four hours. Write down, on separate lines, up to five things you are grateful or thankful for. Common ones include "waking up this morning," "wonderful parents," "good friends," "Self-Health." Do this every night for ten days and see if you don't notice a difference in your stress, anxiety, appreciation, gratitude, and, soon thereafter, your Self-Health. You can get started with your very own Gratitude Journal now. We have some cool ones to choose from on our website.

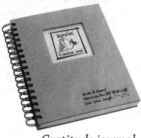

Gratitude journal.

Counting Sheep: America's Pastime

How well do you sleep? You can't really talk about diseases of the heart without talking about sleep. In fact, bitterness, unforgiveness, ingratitude, worry, and stress wreak havoc on our sleeping patterns.

One of the side effects of curing yourself of the diseases of the heart is that you will sleep better. Deep sleep is perhaps the Holy Grail of health. Many seek it, but few find it. Most Americans today sleep 25 percent less than our great-grandparents did. Forty percent of us don't come close to getting the minimum seven hours of sleep that we need for optimal health, and a whopping 20 percent of us get less than six hours of sleep nightly. It's gotten so bad in the United States that we now have a National Sleep Awareness Week. Sponsored by guess who? That's right: Our friends in the pharmaceutical industry.

Luna Moths in Little Kids' Bedrooms

Have you seen the butterfly in your bedroom? It's actually a moth, a luna moth, to be exact—the beautiful, green, sleep-inducing Lunesta luna moth. Fifty million people invited that moth into their bedroom in 2011, and that number is growing rapidly every year.

It's not just the adults the drug companies are after. Would you believe they are now marketing sleeping pills to kids to help them rest up for school? Drug companies recently ran ads that showed images of children, chalkboards, and school buses. The commercial said, "Rozerem would like to remind you that it's back-to-school season. Ask your doctor today if Rozerem is right for you."

The Sleeping Pill Nightmare

Not surprisingly, we are now discovering that the lovely luna moth is not as helpful as we imagined and its effects are not the stuff of dreams. More like nightmares. Studies show that once you start taking sleeping pills, you may need more and more of the drug to get the same effect, and you may not be able to sleep without it. If you try to stop taking sleep medication, you could have withdrawal symptoms (nausea, sweating, and shaking) or what they call "rebound insomnia." As you can imagine, it's worse than the insomnia you had before you met the moth. In his revealing book, *The Dark Side of Sleeping Pills,* Dr. Daniel F. Kripke presents research that shows sleeping pills can shorten the life span, lower immunity to disease, increase the risk of cancer, and cause sudden death.

As the blockbuster Batman movie recently opened, I am reminded of the tragic and unnecessary death of the hugely talented young actor Heath Ledger, who died, perhaps, simply trying to get a good night's sleep. Ironically, the murder suspect in the horrific Aurora, Colorado, theater massacre is reported to have allegedly had the same drug in his system. That's a massive price to pay for a pill that only puts you to sleep seven to sixteen minutes faster than a sugar pill will and

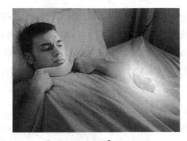

Lunesta nightmare.

increases total sleep time only eleven to nineteen minutes, according to a study conducted in 2011.

Although pills are not the answer, if we are not getting our sleep, we could be putting our Self-Health in serious jeopardy.

The Downside of Sleep Deprivation

What happens when we don't get our Zs? It may surprise you. Sleep deprivation can alter your stress hormones, cause weight gain (you eat more when you're tired), raise blood sugar, put you at risk for diabetes, lower your immune system, affect your heart rate, lead to depression and loss of memory, and even cause brain damage. Lack of sleep can also kill you instantly by way of a car accident: each year 71,000 people are killed because the driver fell asleep at the wheel. People who sleep deeply seven hours a night actually live longer.

The brain, your body's internal doctor, doesn't go to sleep at night; it actually works at the same or higher metabolic level as when you are awake. During sleep, your brain, which pays attention to the outside world during the day, goes to work on healing and repairing the inside world: your core temperature drops, conserving energy; deep breathing increases oxygen flow; and in-flight entertainment begins, in the form of dreams.

Your brain has only a few hours to repair, rebuild, replace, and restore body cells that have worked hard all day and are worn out (one billion cells a day). If you are not sleeping deeply or as long as you should, there's no telling how negatively this healing process is being affected.

Foods That Improve Your Snooze

There are several foods that will improve your snooze. Some foods are rich in tryptophan, an amino acid that the body uses to make its own sleeping drugs (serotonin and melatonin), which in turn slows down nerve traffic and puts you to sleep so the brain can focus on healing activities. Foods that are high in tryptophan are bananas, dark chocolate (75 percent cacao or more), whole wheat grains, organic peanut butter, mushrooms (especially portabella, porcini, and chanterelle), cashews, Brazil nuts, pumpkin seeds, sunflower seeds, pecans, dried figs, dried dates, dried papaya, dried pine-

apple, watermelon, cherries, and celery. Some supplements that can also help are melatonin (the body's natural sleeping potion), valerian (an herb used for centuries to treat insomnia), and magnesium and calcium, which relax your muscles. The powdered form of magnesium and calcium is best. I use Ionic-Fizz Magnesium Plus to help me relax. You can find Ionic-Fizz at your local health food store or on our website, www.SelfHealthRevolution.com.

Foods That Keep You Up at Night

When it comes to sleeping well at night, what you don't eat could be more important than what you do eat. There are some foods that will definitely keep you counting sheep at night.

Caffeine is a stimulant. If you plan to go to bed at 11, you need to stop your caffeine intake by 3. It takes about eight hours for the liver to break down caffeine and eliminate it.

Unless you're passed out drunk, **alcohol** will not let you sleep through the night. Alcohol seems relaxing at first, but it interferes with your brain's production of serotonin (a sleeping drug) and will wake you back up after a few hours of sleeping.

Artificial sweeteners are worse than sugar and will keep you up all night. Aspartame and NutraSweet contain chemicals that excite the nervous system.

Various **prescription and over-the-counter medications**, cold remedies, diuretics, stimulants, and weight-loss products, such as Extra Strength Excedrin, Dexatrim, Vanquish, and Dristan, will rob you of sleep. These all contain high doses of caffeine.

For a free list of foods that make you snooze and foods that make you lose (sleep), check our website.

Secrets to Fighting Insomnia

If there is a silver bullet for insomnia, it's likely to be exercise. Exercising each day for fifteen minutes or longer will actually do more to boost serotonin in your body than anything else you can do. When you come down off your aerobic high some four to eight hours later, your body naturally craves sleep.

Your bedroom temperature should be 65 to 75 degrees and should be as dark as possible. Invest in a comfortable bed, pillow, and sheets. Avoid overstimulation from watching TV or anything that might cause heightened emotions. Calm yourself with positive thoughts and memories. Inhale deeply and exhale slowly; this will slow down your heart rate and relax you. Listen to mellow music or sounds, make an entry or read through your Gratitude Journal, watch a comforting video, or listen to a relaxing speaker. Surround yourself with sleepy smells. A little lavender on the pillow has been proven to help.

You must find a way to sleep and sleep well if you are going to be successful at Self-Health. For the next ten days focus on getting at least seven hours of sleep each night. Don't let anything stop you. See how much better you feel. This could be your most important Self-Health discovery yet.

By now you know a lot of what you didn't know before you started reading this book. There's much more to learn from the book, our website, and a thousand other sources you will discover on your Self-Health journey. Sure, you don't know everything, but you know enough. It's time now for you to begin your Self-Health Revolution. Are you ready to get started? Do you realize that your life is never going to be the same? I wonder how many people you will impact with your own personal Self-Health Revolution?

Self-Health Summary: The Ten-Day Challenge

5 Things Your Body Must Have Every Day (from chapter 10)

FEVPO = Fruits (Eat widely)
Enzymes (Broad spectrum)
Vegetables (Eat widely)
Probiotics (Broad spectrum)
Oils (Pristine source)

2 Things You Must Do Every Day to Get FEVPO (from chapter 10)

- 15 Minute Self-Health Smoothie (recipe in chapter 15)
- 15 Minute Self-Health Salad (recipe in chapter 15)

Next Self-Health Steps (from chapter 11)

- Living H_2O (drink half your weight in ounces of alkaline water)
- Living O_2 (start with 15 minutes of walking and deep breathing every day)

More Mental and Spiritual Self-Health Steps

- Argue with Your ANTs (dispute negative thoughts and replace them with positive ones)
- Give the gift of forgiveness (REACH)
- Practice gratitude (write down five things you're thankful for daily in your Gratitude Journal)
- Get seven hours of deep, restful sleep daily (use Self-Health insomnia secrets)

CHAPTER FOURTEEN

Start a Revolution

Many people die with their music still in them. Why is this so? Too often it is because they are always getting ready to live. Before they know it, time runs out.
—Oliver Wendell Holmes, former U.S. Supreme Court justice

One out of 100 Billion

This Self-Health Revolution is about you. It's about taking control of your life, your heart, and your health and becoming the person that you have always dreamed of being and were created to be. Think about it. Out of the roughly 7 billion people who are alive today and out of 100 billion people who have ever lived, you are undeniably unique. You are not an accident, nor are you incidental. In all of history there has never been anyone exactly like you. No one can duplicate your DNA. You are truly one of a kind. One out of 100 billon, to be exact.

You are a work of art created by God himself. You're not a mass-produced product from some assembly line. You were deliberately planned, created by the heavens as a gift to give the world. You have a song to sing that only you can sing, a symphony to compose that only you can write, a divine musical score that the world needs to hear. Self-Health is about making the commitment to sing your song, write your symphony, and play your music while you can. It's about deciding you will not die with your destiny unrealized and your music still in you.

Self-Health is also about helping others. This book is my sincere attempt to help you. I have poured out my heart after hours of research, study, contem-

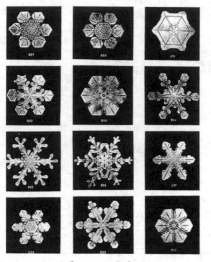

*Like snowflakes,
no two people are alike.*

plation, and even a few tears because I want you to know what I have learned and how it has changed my life. I deeply want it to change your life too and, more than anything else, change the lives of thousands and perhaps millions who might hear this message through you.

Some Things Have to Be Believed to Be Seen

It may sound idealistic and naïve, but what if we could wake this nation up and get everyone to reclaim their Self-Health? What if we could convince them to stop eating fake foods, to question their doctors, to say *no* to drugs and *yes* to living foods? What if the average American knew the things that

you now know? What could happen for those children who are presently destined for diabetes, obesity, and drugs? What could happen to those millions of people who in the next five years will go in for a regular checkup only to find out that they have cancer or heart disease? What could happen to your family and your friends if they knew what you now know? How many lives could we save? How many destinies would be forever altered? Do you think it's possible to make a difference?

Imagine it. Fathers live to see their daughter's wedding. Mothers get to hug their grandkids. Children would no longer have to stand over the graves of their heroes. Imagine people of all walks of life putting down their drugs, pushing away fake foods, eating to live, happy and healthy, living life to the fullest, feeling fit, full of energy, getting older without aging, living to be a ripe old age, free of pain, chronic illnesses, doctors, hospitals, and pharmaceuticals. Is this an impossible dream? Sometimes things have to be believed to be seen.

I am a dreamer, but not altogether naïve. I realize that we cannot rid the world of sickness, sorrow, disease, and pain. But if we truly believe that giving our bodies what they so desperately need will heal our self-inflicted wounds, then doesn't it stand to reason that sharing this knowledge with those we love could dramatically change their lives? And as we share, more people will be awakened and in turn share the knowledge of Self-Health with others, exponentially increasing the sphere of impact.

It Has Happened Before, and It Can Happen Again

Perhaps it starts with one person, who tells another person; they grow into a few, a few becomes a group, a group becomes a crowd, a crowd becomes a mass, a mass gives birth to a movement, and a movement turns into a revolution. There was a time when twelve Jewish fishermen and a lowly carpenter turned the world upside down in one generation. A French nineteen-year-old peasant girl named Joan once bravely raised a homemade flag and repelled the armies of England, reclaiming her homeland for all time. A short, balding, tired, old Indian named Gandhi broke the bonds of English tyranny and freed his people from the most powerful nation of that era. A humble, middle-aged housekeeper named Rosa Parks refused to give up her seat on a bus and sparked a movement that has brought freedom and equality to millions of people and now our first Black American president. These are only a few of the thousands of examples that I could recite. My point is a simple one: If it has happened before, it can happen again.

A Secret You Should Share

This Self-Health Revolution is not about money, fame, power, or success. I'm not out to be the next health food guru or another Tony Robbins. This revolution is about helping people and changing lives. The hero here is the power of this information and the message of Self-Health. Read this book, put it to the test, try the Self-Health lifestyle for ten days, put these

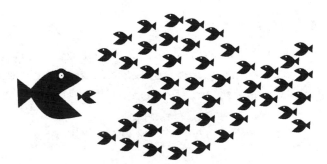

There are more of us than there are of them.

teachings into practice, and if you get results, if it changes your life, then join our Self-Health Revolution. Don't keep a great secret to yourself. Tell people you know and love. They need this message. Share the book. Visit our website. Sign up for our newsletters and videos. Come to our seminars and bring the people you love. They desperately need to know about the secret of Self-Health.

In many ways the success of the Self-Health Revolution is not within my power. I am trusting in you. In the end, you will determine whether we win or lose this battle against the greedy, dark elements of our society who put profits before people, money over morals, and cash above cures. They will undoubtedly win if we don't act. Who knows how much worse it will become for our children and our children's children. So test us, try us, and then join us, and together we will be the ones who do something to save ourselves and start the Self-Health Revolution.

No Self-Health Guru Here

I want to thank you for caring enough about yourself and your loved ones to take time to read this book. As I sit here writing the last words of this long letter after many days, I feel that I have come to know you and hope you feel that you know a little about me too. I am truly nothing great. I have fears, weaknesses, and shortcomings, and I make mistakes like everyone else.

The power and truth of this book do not rest on me, my credentials, or the thousands of people who have contributed their wisdom about Self-Health directly or indirectly. The strength of this message comes from eternal truths handed down through the ages, of which I am an unworthy messenger. These are teachings that even our own hearts tell us are true.

Ultimately you have within yourself the power to prove the message to be true or false. My prayer for you is that you will indeed find your Self-Health

---

I am only one, but still I am one. I cannot do everything, but still I can do something; and because I cannot do everything I will not refuse to do the something that I can do.

—EDWARD EVERETT HALE,
AMERICAN AUTHOR AND THEOLOGIAN

and share that message with as many as possible. If we meet here on Earth or in some celestial place, I hope you can say that I have made a difference in your life and that you would count me as your friend.

Please feel free to contact me with comments, questions, ideas, or testimonials: JMichaelZenn@gmail.com.

Self-Health Is In Your Hands

An ancient story is told of an old Chinese wise man with a long, white beard living high in the mountains. He was renowned throughout the kingdom for his wisdom. One day two young boys decided to put the old man's wisdom to the test. They caught a small bird in the forest and made the several days' climb up the mountain in search of the old wise man. When they found him, they boldly stood before him and said, "Behind our backs, we hold a small bird in our hands. Tell us, in your great wisdom, is the bird dead or alive?"

The old man knelt on the ground and began to write something in the sand with his finger. Drawing on his wisdom, he knew that if he said the bird was dead, the boys would open their hands and let the bird fly away. If he said the bird was alive, they would squeeze their hands and bring its life to an end.

The old man looked down at the ground for a few more minutes, then slowly raised his head and said, "Whether the bird lives or whether the bird dies is not for me to say. You see, my sons, the fate of this little bird does not rest with me; its fate lies within your hands."

Self-Health is now in your hands. I trust you will keep it alive.

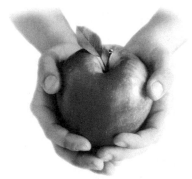

CHAPTER FIFTEEN

Self-Health Recipes

It's time to start living the life you've imagined.
—Henry James

Three Years of Proven Results

The following are recipes that I have developed over three years of personal testing and proven results. I use most of them on a daily basis. They are delicious, powerful, and the foundation of my own Self-Health. Each recipe is packed with more plant chemicals and nutrients than most people see in months or even years of eating. With most of them I have included a quick, simple version and a more powerful version that you can start with or grow into if you choose.

Be Flexible

I suggest you use organic ingredients as much as possible, but I understand that some organic foods may be too expensive or not available in your area. These recipes are not rigid. If there is an ingredient you do not like, then simply replace it with something else. Over time these recipes will evolve into your own. I'm sure you will discover even better combinations. I hope you will share your discoveries with me so the Self-Health team can share your culinary secrets with future readers. I'll be happy to acknowledge your contribution in our newsletter or on the website. Our website has printable copies of all recipes, plus even more recipes, and you can sign up for a sneak preview of *The Self Health Revolution Cookbook*, coming soon.

Self-Health Tools

The only Self-Health tools you will need to get started are a blender, a good vegetable peeler, a tea or coffee brewer, Ziploc bags, Glad Press'n Seal plastic wrap, and a very large salad bowl. My favorite blenders are Vitamix and BlendTec. They cost more but last forever and blend just about anything. Check our web-site for info.

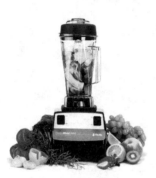

Vitamix blender.

Smoothie and Salad Before Anything Else

Drink the Self-Health Smoothie as soon as you rise in the morning. Do this before you go to work and prior to eating anything else. The Self-Health Salad is great for lunch and as a dinner entrée with your favorite wild-caught fish, tofu, or free-range, grass-fed beef or chicken. Choose your own salad dressing. Try to stay healthy in your choice of dressing, but this is an area where I splurge a little. Just don't go crazy. Again, eat these salads for lunch and dinner before you eat anything else. Eat as much of the salad as you want. Once you get hooked on these living foods, nothing else will compare. Don't worry if you miss a day. Just get right back to your Self-Health Smoothie and Salad as soon as you can.

Fifteen-Minute Self-Health Smoothie (serves 1–2)

Blend the following ingredients on high for one minute. Pour into a large glass and drink to your Self-Health. If traveling to the office or work, be sure to get a large portable cup and sip on this delicious smoothie throughout the morning. Remember, if there is an ingredient that you do not like, simply replace it with something you like better. Drink this smoothie before eating anything else. (If raspberries and blackberries are not available, substitute blueberries and strawberries. Frozen is okay too, especially if harvested wild. Use frozen berries if you like your smoothie more frosty.)

1 cup of blueberries
1 cup strawberries
½ cup raspberries
½ cup blackberries
1 banana
1 powder pack of Nature's Way Primadophilus Intensive
    Probiotic (or crack open one capsule and add the powder
    to the mix)
2 tablespoons Nordic Naturals or Carlson's omega-3 fish oil
1 to 2 scoops Vibrant Health Green Vibrance powder
¼ cup whole leaf Lily of the Desert aloe vera gel (Inner Fillet
    only)
1½ cups not-from-concentrate orange or apple juice
2 ounces green tea (You can use leftover tea leaves from
    the pot.)
1 to 2 teaspoons raw dark honey to taste

Self-Health Super Smoothie (serves 2–3)

If raspberries and blackberries are not available, substitute blueberries and strawberries. Frozen is okay too, especially if harvested wild.

½ cup of blueberries
½ cup strawberries
½ cup raspberries
½ cup blackberries
½ mango peeled and cut
½ organic kiwi peeled
½ apricot peeled
½ cup cherries deseeded
½ cup freshly cut pineapple
½ banana
1 broken capsule of Nature's Way Primadophilus Probiotic
2 tablespoons Nordic Naturals or Carlson's omega-3 fish oil
2 scoops Vibrant Health Green Vibrance powder
¼ cup whole leaf Lily of the Desert aloe vera gel (Inner Fillet only)
¼ cup not-from-concentrate black cherry juice
¼ cup not-from-concentrate pomegranate juice
¼ cup not-from-concentrate grape juice
¼ cup not-from-concentrate cranberry juice
¼ cup not-from-concentrate orange or apple juice
20 drops organic clove extract (HerbPharm)
2 ounces green tea (You can use leftover tea leaves from the pot.)
1 to 2 teaspoons raw dark honey to taste

For Ultra-Self-Health Smoothie, add Genesis Fusion 4 (Goji, Acai, Noni, Mangosteen).

Self-Health Fifteen-Minute Salad Mix (8–10 servings)

Simply toss the following ingredients into a very large salad bowl and mix thoroughly. Glad Press'n Seal makes a great reusable cover for a large bowl. You will use this mix as your source of salad for the next several days. To take to work, put your salad in a bowl or a Ziploc bag with your dressing on the side. I eat this fantastic salad twice a day before I eat anything else—once at lunch and once at dinner.

    5-ounce box organic Earthbound Farms Fresh Herb Salad
    5-ounce box organic Earthbound Farms Baby Spinach
    5-ounce box organic Earthbound Farms Baby Arugula
    10-ounce pack organic sweet grape or cherry tomatoes
    12 ounces organic precut broccoli, carrots, and cauliflower

Self-Health Super Salad Mix (10–12 servings)

Add these ingredients to Self-Health Fifteen-Minute Salad Mix.

> 4-ounce pack of broccoli sprouts (BroccoSprouts brand) or Brocco Sprouts Salad Blend (broccoli, clover, and radish sprouts)
> ¼-ounce pack of organic mint (plucked)
> ¼-ounce pack of organic basil (plucked)
> ¼-ounce pack of finely chopped organic rosemary
> 5-ounce bunch chopped fresh cilantro

Want to take your Self-Health even higher? Spruce up your individual salad with chopped onions, peppers (yellow, red, orange, white), cucumbers, mushrooms, and asparagus.

Take it up another nutritional notch from there with chopped radishes, okra, sweet potatoes, beet root (yellow and red), celery root, ginger root, and turmeric root. If you juice vegetables, save your leftovers in a Ziploc bag and spread them over your individual salads to boost your Self-Health.

Kick Tail Tea

Kick Tail Tea is something you can start drinking in the morning and drink all day until around 3 so that it doesn't interfere with sleep. It's a great replacement for coffee, and as its name suggests, it does kick tail. You will feel a smooth flow of energy and mental clarity all day long. If you don't have the money to buy the whole leaf loose leaf teas, you can get less expensive brands like Numi at Whole Foods Market or a health food store or grocer near by. The important thing is to get the full spectrum of the different teas in your body daily. Each tea has unique chemicals that boost your body in different ways. The premium recipe is simply the most powerful tea that you can find anywhere. If you try it, you will see what I mean. I drink a pot daily.

Self-Health Kick Tail Green Tea

Mix together loose tea in a container and store. Use two teabags or teaspoons per one cup of water. To prepare, brew until water temperature is around 140 degrees or just slightly too hot to touch. Do not boil or overheat your tea, or you will destroy the enzymes and nutrients you are seeking. Allow the bags or loose tea to remain in the pot for richer and more powerful tea. If you are like me and more adventurous about your Self-Health, drink your tea totally unfiltered and chew on your tea leaves to get even more plant nutrients. Drink one to four cups daily.

BUDGET MIX
- White tea
- Green tea
- Green Rooibos Tea
- Chai tea
- Oolong tea

PREMIUM MIX
- Republic of Tea Full-Leaf Loose Tea
- Silver Rain White Tea
- Golden Yunan Black Tea
- Milk Oolong Tea
- Dancing Leaves Green Tea
- Organic Raw Green Bush Rooibos
- Matcha Green (not full leaf)

Mega Trail Mix

The Mega Trail Mix is an unbelievably powerful snack that you can munch on throughout the day and even in the evening. Because the mix is so dense, you may want to eat only a few ounces at a time. It can also be a good replacement for dessert and a good way to squelch food cravings. Compare the ingredients with any trail mix on the market and you will find that it blows them out of the water.

Self-Health Mega Trail Mix *(10–12 servings)*

Mix the following ingredients and store in a large double-bagged Ziploc to maintain freshness.

2 cups raw sunflower seeds
1 cup raw pumpkin seeds
1 cup raw Brazil nuts
1 cup raw almonds
½ cup raw flaxseed
1 cup dried goji berries
1 cup dried cherries
1 cup dried raisins
1 cup dried cranberries
½ cup dried apricots
½ cup dried prunes

Three-Pepper Guacamole

The Three-Pepper Guacamole is one of the best-tasting dips ever. It's all raw food, packed with nutrients, and a great recipe for entertaining and introducing new people to living foods. You can use it as a dip or spread it over wild-caught fish, organic eggs, blackened tofu, grilled grass-fed steak or chicken. If you eat it as a dip, I suggest using organic blue corn chips. Garden of Eatin' is a great brand that I like a lot. I make this awesome dish two or three times a week.

Self-Health Three-Pepper Guacamole

Mix the following ingredients in a large bowl. Leave the avocado seeds in the mix. (It keeps avocadoes fresh longer.) Use as a dip, a topping, or a sauce. Eat as dip with organic blue corn chips. Store in Ziploc bag to take to work or to save as a snack for later.

    3 ripe organic avocadoes, diced
    ½ chopped red onion
    1 5-ounce bunch cilantro, chopped
    1 large or 2 small celery stalks, chopped fine
    1 10-once pack of organic sweet cherry tomatoes
    4 cloves of fresh garlic, pressed
    ⅛ cup fresh squeezed lime juice
    1 to 2 tablespoons raw dark honey to taste
    1 teaspoon fresh ground peppercorns
    1 teaspoon Lawry's Seasoned Salt (or generic seasoning salt)
    1 teaspoon Tabasco Garlic Pepper Sauce (or pepper sauce)
    2 fresh serrano peppers, chopped fine
    1 yellow chili, chopped fine
    1 small fresh jalapeño chili, chopped fine (add to taste)
    Pinch of curry (add to taste)

What Are the Living Foods on Your Plate?

It is important to get as much living food into your body as possible. Look at your plate. How much living food is there? Look at the menu. What living foods are on the menu? Make sure you are eating at least 80 percent living foods. If you are going to eat some-thing dead, then eat your living foods first and limit your dead foods to 20 percent of what you eat.

Have fun with living foods. Discover new recipes that excite you. Become a food alchemist and create formulas of your own. Remember, variety is the spice of life and the key to your health, so include as many ingredients as possible.

CHAPTER 16

The Self-Health Revolutioneers

*It's time to wake up and live the life
you have always dreamed of*

Two Friends at Work and 100 Pounds: Rosetta Fraleigh and Tracy Davis Harmon

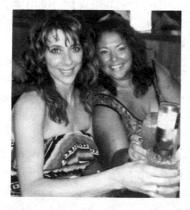

Rosetta's Story

I am a very busy mother, wife, and successful entrepreneur. I own and run a wonderful business, where I employ fourteen women. A few months ago I found myself looking in the mirror and not liking the image I saw staring back at me. I was not obese but very overweight. Although I hid it well, I was really unhappy with myself. A friend of mine handed me a book and said that I might be ready to read it. The book was *The Self-Health Revolution*. I read it, and I finally got it! I decided to take the ten-day challenge. It changed my life.

That night, after my son refused to eat what I thought at the time was a healthful meal, I lost it and threw out all the junk food in my home. I went to the grocery store and filled my refrigerator and pantry with wonderful fresh, living foods, the kind that I had grown up with. It finally made sense: If I feed my body what it needs, then I won't be hungry. I fell in love with all kinds of wonderful vegetables and greens. Unbelievably, just as it said in the book, I started craving these incredible nutritious foods, and my appetite for sweets, sugars, and junk food faded and almost disappeared. The weight fell off, seemingly without effort. My mom always told me that I couldn't lose weight without exercise (she was a marathon runner), but this time I proved her wrong.

In ten weeks I had lost forty pounds! I weigh less now than I did on my wedding day. There are no words to express my gratitude and thanks to Mr. Zenn and his book. Some of my relatives couldn't believe how fast I was losing weight and thought something must be wrong with me. The women at my company began to notice my new energy and great new figure. They all wanted to know what diet I was on. I told them, "It's not a diet. It's a whole new way of thinking about food." They wanted to know more, so I started telling my story and handing out books. I must have given out twenty books. One of the people I gave the book to was my very sweet but skeptical friend of fifteen years, Tracy Harmon. She was on a diet, but like so many diets it was very difficult to follow and it wasn't really working for her.

Tracy's Story

I noticed my friend and coworker Rosetta was really losing weight and looking and feeling great. All of us at the office were wondering, "What was she doing?" We thought she was on some new diet. I myself was on a diet and trying to lose weight, so I asked her. She told me about a book she had read, *The Self-Health Revolution*, and how it was helping her lose weight like mad and how she felt so amazing. Of course, I was very skeptical, and I took what she said with a grain of salt. I even worried that she wasn't healthy. It all seemed too fast and just too easy. She had watched me struggle with my weight, measuring and counting and being hungry, frustrated, and falling off the diet wagon over and over again. I had reached a point in my life where I was ill physically and mentally, depressed, and just overall felt terrible in my own skin. So knowing me as she does she said, "You are the most stubborn person I know. Just read the book and take something from it, even if it is just one thing."

I thought all this eating living food stuff was not for me. I loved my soda. I knew I could lose weight only by measuring and weighing and being strict. But she was so excited and happy that I said, What the heck!

This book was an absolute eye-opener. I decided I would give it a try and started with the smoothie. I am now 54 pounds lighter, and I swear I feel better at forty years old than I have in longer than I can remember! Eating living food is even easier than picking up fast food. I don't count. I don't measure. I eat when I am hungry, and my taste buds are fascinated at how good food tastes again. I vacation and still lose weight. I don't crave my bad foods like I used to, and when I do, I figure out how to eat something better and more healthful. Rosetta came up with an awesome protein scone recipe, and now the whole office is addicted.

People around me have said, "Wow! Whatever it is you are doing, it agrees with you. Keep it up. It is so nice to see you looking so at ease and happy." I still have more weight to lose, but it feels different this time. I know it is not a sprint; it is a marathon. And I am not only going to complete it, but I will win! In fact, I am winning for the first time I can remember.

My friend Rosetta and I tell anyone who will listen about the Self-Health Revolution and the amazing change it has created in our lives. So please, read the book, get on the ten-day challenge, and take something from it, even if it is only one thing. Just one thing can change your life!

A Real Southerner: Rickey Pittman, Author, Storyteller, and Folksinger

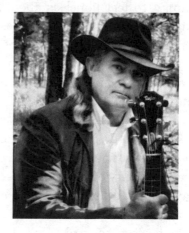

I consider myself just an average, regular guy, born and bred in the South. I am certainly not a health nut and have never shopped at Whole Foods, nor have my friends or family. I pretty much ate the traditional diet that my parents and grandparents, who also grew up in the South, ate. I couldn't figure out why, year after year, I seemed to be getting sicker and fatter, along with most of my friends and relatives. I truly did not realize how much food had changed over the past couple of decades.

A few months ago I was lucky enough to receive as a gift J. Michael Zenn's book, *The Self-Health Revolution*, and it has forever changed my whole perspective on food, dieting, and health. I had quit smoking a few years ago. The year I quit smoking, I gained about

40 pounds and found myself on blood pressure and cholesterol medication. Needless to say, I was depressed and beginning to feel hopeless about my new fat self. I was raised on processed foods and the fried, fatty foods of the South. I had thought myself invincible and not susceptible to the ravages of middle age and an undisciplined lifestyle. I read Michael's book, and wow, it woke me up. I realized, right then, I needed a revolution.

The simplicity of his commonsense suggestions and the logic of his message made so much sense. I began to cut out most of the bad "dead" foods, drinking more and better water, exercising more, eating as close to "natural" (living) foods as I could, and as a result and seemingly without effort, I have already dropped down from a 40 waist to a 36 and am well on my way to a 32. I never thought my pants sizes would go backward. My energy has increased.

I still have a ways to go, but I intend to follow through with the only health plan I've found that made sense and that can be adapted to my lifestyle and a career that has me constantly on the road. As an author and avid reader, I've perused many books on health and dieting, but this is the only one I would recommend to others. Funny, I still don't consider myself to be a health nut, but I have definitely begun my own Self-Health Revolution!

A Star Athlete: Tim Thigpen

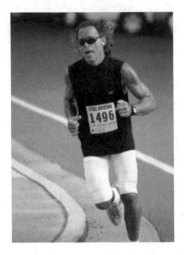

Some people have always been able to eat whatever they please. Either they were the lucky ones who never put on weight, or they simply burn off the calories by exercising. I was in the latter category.

Playing high school sports and then college tennis kept me fit and ready to take on the professional world when I graduated. The one exercise I never stopped doing was running. From 1979, when I finished college, to 2008, I ran several times a week (many weeks I ran every day), and I ate anything I pleased. Fast, processed, and inexpensive food items like chicken wings made me happy. Quite frankly, organic food was a little scary!

I was at Lake Lanier Resort near Atlanta for a weekend vacation when Michael Zenn came for a Sunday afternoon by the pool. All he would talk about was his health and nutrition quest and "living food." I could not get him off the subject. "Do you know how little nutrition is in farm-raised salmon? Do you know what actually is in margarine?" And "Pringles are not real food!" When I ordered some mango-habanera wings from the pool-side bar, he looked at me and said, "Would you like to hear about growth hormone side effects?"

Honestly, I thought Michael had gone too far, but he convinced me to put his beliefs to the test. "Okay," I said, "I will read the book, and I will take your ten-day challenge. I promise I will begin tomorrow with an organic, wild-caught, no-processed foods, blah, blah, blah diet. I mean nutrition plan. And we will see." My first thought was that, because I ran most days, and more specifically, because for the past few years I raced in 5Ks, 10Ks, half-marathons, and marathons, I had a perfect benchmark of any impact this nutrition change would or would not have on me and my performance. My second thought was, "How is this food going to taste?" My perspective was how bad light and reduced-calorie food tasted, or rather, did *not* taste! The thought of being younger, stronger, and faster interested me, for sure, but what was I going to have to eat to do it, and would it really work?

It was at that moment Zenn reached into his bag of goodies and broke out some dip he called Three-Pepper Guacamole (a recipe in this book). It was a raw (living foods) conglomeration of different-color peppers, onions, avocados, tomatoes, honey, and so forth with the amazing smell of cilantro. One taste and WOW, I was hooked! I went home and read *The Self-Health Revolution*, and for almost four years now, WOW happens every day! Not only did I see clear and measurable performance results that I can share with you, but I simply fell in love with the Self-Health food and lifestyle.

I was also shocked to read the story in Zenn's book of how Jim Fixx, the father of modern running, although he ran five miles a day, dropped dead of a massive heart attack because of his diet. I realized then that I could be fit but not healthy at all. It also excited me to read about how, in some cultures, runners and athletes actually got better, stronger, and faster as they age because of their diet.

Here are the things I immediately began to experience (or not experience):

No STUFFED feelings
No HUNGER feelings
No CRAVING for bad food (wings, etc.)
No MEDICATIONS
No SICKNESS
No NEED A NAP in the afternoon feeling

The most amazing bathroom
experiences
No need for the little blue pill (you
can figure this one out)

But let's really put this to the test!
When I was growing up, my grandmother and mother made sure I started
my day with a pot of coffee, just as they
did. I love coffee, have come to depend
on it, and have never attempted to go
cold turkey on my morning caffeine
injection. Would this new living food
I was eating replace the boost I was
getting every morning from my coffee
fix? Could I do this for a month, I won-
dered, and what would be the effects?
So, for one month, no coffee touched
my lips. I had a glass of Self-Health
Smoothie and living foods every morn-

ing and never noticed any difference or
difficulty. In fact, I had more energy
than ever.

I realize that everything I am saying
can be said by anyone, whether it's true
or not. Many people on TV commercials claim these same results. However, what I will tell you next cannot be
made up.

Even though I have been an avid
runner most of my life and during
my early forties started running com-
petitive local races, I am much faster
now in my mid-fifties than I ever was
in my mid-forties. And the *only thing
I changed* was the Ten-Day Challenge
and Self-Health lifestyle based entirely
on Zenn's *Self-Health Revolution* book.
Here's the proof:

Year	Race	Location	Age	Result/Place
2003	5K Run Downtown	Greenville, SC	45	21:10/Did Not Place
2009	5K Run Downtown	Greenville, SC	51	19:20/1st in Age
2004	5K Grasshopper	Cowpens Battle Field	47	21:55/Did Not Place
2009	5K Grasshopper	Cowpens Battle Field	51	19:11/1st in Age
2005	5K Spinx Run Fest	Greenville, SC	47	21:24/Did Not Place
2010	5K Spinx Run Fest	Greenville, SC	52	19:04/1st in Age
2004	26.2m Philly Marathon	Philadelphia, PA	46	4:10:33
2011	26.2m Thunder Road Mar.	Charlotte, NC	53	3:16:17/Qualified for Boston Marathon

Late in 2010 I started cross-training
on my bike. In 2011, I decided to take
my Self-Health Revolution challenge to

triathlons. In my first year, at age fifty-
four (in the 50–54 Age Group), here are
my Self-Health triathlon results:

Placed 1st in my age group in my
first four triathlons
Ranked in the top three in South
Carolina in my age group
Qualified for and participated
in the U.S. Age Group National
Championships
Earned a ranking in the Top 100 in
my age group in the country

The bottom line is this: When I was sitting by the pool at Lake Lanier, having reached the age of fifty, I was an avid runner and not overweight, but I could not catch my peers. Five years later they cannot catch me. What I changed, and the results that occurred, is found in Zenn's *Self-Health Revolution* book. Because of my results, I am often asked to make presentations and coach athletes around the country to teach how they can actually improve their performance through Self-Health as they get older.

Zenn's Self-Health can have a life-changing impact beyond weight loss and great health. It's unbelievable to me that even in my mid-fifties I am still getting younger, stronger, and faster every single day.

A College Athlete and Medical Student: Mack Lorden

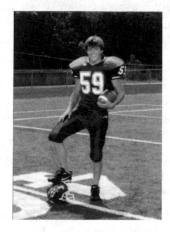

I am an eighteen-year-old college freshman. I am happy to report that *The Self-Health Revolution* seemed to be written just for me. I couldn't put it down.

This letter is a testament to the "Gratitude and Forgiveness" chapter in this book. The book had a profound effect on me and my future. I am now attending Ohio State University, studying medical dietetics. In my high school, I was always very interested in anatomy and chemistry classes. I was also a varsity football captain. But the trait that sets me apart from others is now my Self-Health.

At first it was rough. In high school, every single day I would pack a lunch of fruit and turkey. I was tempted nearly every day by our school's fake food meals and my friends' confused looks and questions, but somehow my discipline and Self-Health held. Not only were my packed lunches healthful, but breakfast and dinner were too. I suppose the reason I began to eat healthfully is that my abs were starting to protrude, and I desperately wanted that eight-pack. (You know how being a teenager and girls go.) I also noticed that I had better endurance than anybody else on the football team because of my heightened nutrition and Self-Health lifestyle.

I am a good student, and I have often thought about medical school and being a doctor or going through pharmaceutical training. Reading the book has not only enlightened me about these industries and professions but also given me hope and guidance about how I can impact and change the future. I realized that I do not want to live by the pill, but by nature and by this powerful lifestyle. Now I want to encourage others to succeed with me. I want to get stronger and healthier each year as I get older.

I knew I had the discipline to remain healthy, but I did not have the wisdom until I read *The Self-Health Revolution*. I learned many things from your book, and I appreciate the time it took you to gather all of that information. I read the ten-day challenge part, and said to myself, "Screw the ten days, I'll try it for life."

By now I'm sure you realize how much the Self-Health Revolution has

influenced my future. I now have a solid grasp on what I want to do with my life. Once again, Mr. Zenn, many thanks. I know that I am not the only one who has found your book a lifesaver. I hope the Self-Health Revolution will continue to thwart the terrible diets, fake foods, and reckless habits of Americans. I firmly believe that this lifestyle can and *will* turn into a revolution. It's only a matter of time. I will join this revolution now and even more positively after I graduate from OSU. Keep fighting, Mr. Zenn, for your sake, and for ours.

A *Teenager and Tennis Player:* Samantha Balanevsky

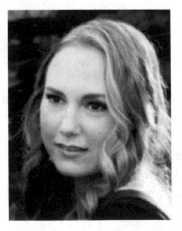

The Self-Health Revolution is one of the most inspiring books I have read. The details and precise explanations in the book showed me this problem from a new perspective. I am a sixteen-year-old girl, and I believe all teenagers should read this book.

I read it in only one day, and it really changed my perspective on this matter. If all teenagers read this book, it could lead to a revolutionary change for health issues in the future.

One dream I have is to end obe-sity in America. I so believe in the Self-Health Revolution that I recently sent a letter and a copy of the book to Michelle Obama because I know she is concerned about changing this obesity epidemic. I believe this book could lead us one step closer to this change.

References

The following books were most helpful. I recommend you obtain them for your personal library. Many of these titles are available on our website, www.SelfHealthRevolution.com.

Bowden, J. (2007). *150 Healthiest Foods on Earth*. Gloucester, MA: Fair Winds Press.

Campbell, T. C. & Campbell, T. M. (2006). *The China Study*. Dallas, TX: Benbella.

Canfield, J. (2005). *The Success Principles*. New York: HarperCollins.

Diamond, H. (2003). *Fit for Life Not Fat for Life*. Deerfield Beach, FL: Health Communication.

Diamond, H. & Diamond, M. (1987). *Fit for Life*. New York: Grand Central.

Fuhrman, J. (2003). *Eat to Live*. Boston: Little, Brown.

Hanley, J. L. & Deville, N. (2001). *Tired of Being Tired*. New York: Berkley.

Hyman, M. & Liponis, M. (2003). *UltraPrevention: The 6-week Plan That Will Make You Healthy for Life*. New York: Atria.

Pollan, M. (2008). *In Defense of Food: An Eater's Manifesto*. New York: Penguin.

Pratt, S. (2007). *SuperFoods Rx*. Emmaus, PA: Rodale Books.

Robbins, A. (1999). *Living Health*. San Diego, CA: Robbins Research International.

Schlosser, E. (2004). *Fast Food Nation: The Dark Side of the All-American Meal*. New York: HarperPerennial.

Seligman, M. E. P. (2002), *Authentic Happiness*. London: Nicholas Brealey Publishing.

Trudeau, K. (2004). *Natural Cures "They" Don't Want You to Know About*. Elk Grove Village, IL: Alliance.

Zucker, M. & Belfield, W. (1981). *How to Have a Healthier Dog*. New York: Doubleday.

Here are some great websites that proved helpful to my research.

AARP, on the numerous benefits of walking, www.AARP.com

Center for Food Safety 2008, www.centerforfoodsafety.org/rbgh_hormo.cfm

Farm Animal Welfare Committee Report, www.fawc.org.uk/reports/pigs/fawcp006.htm

Farm Animal Welfare Council, www.fawc.org.uk/default.htm

Humane Society Press, www.humanesocietypress.org

Harvard Medical School Family Health Guide (on the benefits of taking probiotics), www.health
.harvard.edu/fhg/updates/update0905c.shtml
On nutritional supplements, www.drlwilson.com

**These articles proved helpful to my research. You can find these easily online or through a
good database. For practical purposes, they are listed by article title instead of by author.**

"Agricultural Antibiotic Use Contributes to 'Super-bugs' in Humans." *Science Daily*, July 5, 2005.

"Americans Slightly Taller, Much Heavier Than Four Decades Ago." National Center for Health
Statistics, October 27, 2004.

"Animal Welfare and the Intensification of Animal Production: An Alternative Interpretation." David
Fraser. Food and Agriculture Organization of the United Nations, 2005.

"Antidepressants Most Prescribed Drugs in U.S." Elizabeth Cohen. CDC, July 9, 2007.

"Antidepressants versus Placebos: Meaningful Advantages Are Lacking." Irving Kirsch & David
Antonuccio. *Psychiatric Times*, 2004.

"Associated Press Five Year Study: Drugs Show Up in Americans' Water." Jeff Donn, Martha
Mendoza, & Justin Pritchard. March 10, 2008. Associated Press.

"Baby Food." Andrew F. Smith. *Oxford Encyclopedia of Food and Drink in America*, vol. 1. New York:
Oxford University Press, 2004.

"Bleaching Agent in Flour Linked to Diabetes." Janet Hull. *Idaho Observer*, July 2005.

"Brain Malfunction Explains Dehydration in Elderly." *Science Daily*, December 18, 2007.

"Breathing for Perfect Health: The 3-Season Diet." John Douillard. New York: Three Rivers Press,
2001.

"Bullying of Doctors Alleged at Vioxx Trial." *North Jersey Record*, July 15, 2005.

"Can't Get to Sleep? Try Exercise in the Late Afternoon." Michael J. Breus. *Huffington Post*, July 9,
2008.

"Cattle Feed Is Often a Sum of Animal Parts." Lewis Kamb. *Seattle Post-Intelligencer*, January 28,
2004.

"Cholesterol Drugs and Children: A Recommendation Draws Fire." Tara Parker-Pope. *International
Herald Tribune / New York Times*, July 9, 2008.

"The Claim: Brown Sugar Is Healthier Than White Sugar." Anahad O'Connor. *New York Times*, June
12, 2007.

"Coke, Pepsi Lose Fight over Labels." *Knight Ridder News*, December 9, 2004.

"Concentrated Animal Feeding Operations." CDC, USDHHS, 2011.

"Confessions of a Lymphomaniac." Hugh O'Neill. *Men's Health*, 2008.

"Counting Blessings versus Burdens: An Experimental Investigation of Gratitude and Subjective
Well-being in Daily Life." R. A. Emmons & M. E. McCullough. *Journal of Personality and Social
Psychology* 84 (2003), 377–89.

"Cruelty to Animals: Mechanized Madness." PETA, 2008.

"The Dark Side of Recycling." Keith Woods. *Earth Island Journal*, Fall 1990.

"The Dark Side of Sleeping Pills." Daniel F. Kripke. Self published, 2008, revised February 2012.

"Demand for Animal Products May Double in 20 years." VOA, October 16, 2007.

"Everything You Never Learned About Birds." Rebecca Rupp. Storey Publishing, 1995.

"ExxonMobil Amasses Record $36B 2005 Profit." David J. Lynch. *USA Today*, 2005.

"Factory Farming." *Encyclopaedia Britannica*. Chicago: Encyclopaedia Britannica, Inc., 2007.

"Factory Farming in the Developing World." Danielle Nierenberg. *World Watch Magazine*, May/June
2003.

"Factory Farming: The True Costs." Humane Farming Association. HFA.org, 2008.

"Factory Farms Are Responsible for Bird Flu, According to a New Report." *NF News*, February 20, 2007.

"Factory Farms: The Only Answer to Our Growing Appetite?" Stanley Baker. *The Guardian*, December 29, 1964.

"Facts about Pollution from Livestock Farms." Natural Resources Defense Council. 2006.

"Fact Sheet #1: A Brief History and Background of the EPA CAFO Rule." John Sweeten et al. MidWest Plan Service, Iowa State University, July 2003.

"FDA Links Antidepressants, Youth Suicide Risk." S. Vedantam. *Washington Post*, February 23, 2004.

"Forgive and Be Well?" Melissa Healy. *Los Angeles Times,* December 31, 2007.

"Happiness Is More Than Chasing Pleasure." Jane Weaver. MSNBC. March 19, 2007.

"Harmful Pesticides Found in Everyday Food Products: Mercer Island Children Tested in Yearlong Study." Andrew Schneider. *Seattle PI Newspaper,* January 30, 2008.

"Head to Head: Intensive Farming." *BBC News.* March 6, 2001.

"The Health Benefits of Happiness." Mark Easton. *BBC News.* May 23, 2006.

"HFCS Is Not 'Natural.'" Lorraine Heller. *FDA Report.* 2008.

"History of the Development of Infant Formulas" and "Infant Formula: Evaluating the Safety of New Ingredients." Food and Nutrition Board.

"Hormones in Water Blamed as More Men Seek Breast Reduction." Sarah-Kate Templeton. *Sunday Times*, July 31, 2005.

"How Dogs and Cats Get Recycled into Pet Food." John Eckhouse. *San Francisco Chronicle*, February 1990.

"An HSUS Report: Welfare Issues with Gestation Crates for Pregnant Sows." Humane Society of the United States. January 6, 2006.

"Infant and Child Nutrition." Kenneth F. Kiple and Kriemhild Coneè Ornelas. *Cambridge World History of Food*, vol. 2. Cambridge: Cambridge University Press, 2000.

"Intense Sweetness Surpasses Cocaine Reward." Magalie Lenoir, Fuschia Serre, Lauriane Cantin, & Serge H. Ahmed. University of Bordeaux, 2007.

"Is Factory Farming Really Cheaper?" *New Scientist*, 1971.

"Is Unhappiness the Real Cause of a Lot of Disease?" Scott Mowbray. *Health Magazine,* March 24, 2008.

"Make Friends with Good Bacteria." Cheryl Redmond. *Natural Health*, March 2002.

"Male Fish Becoming Female: Researchers Worry about Estrogen and Pollutants in the Water." Tom Costello. *NBC News*, November 9, 2004.

"Md. Hog Farm Causing Quite a Stink." *Washington Post*, May 23, 1999.

"Merck More about Profits Than Healing." *USA Today,* July 14, 2005.

"Merck Used 'Dodge Ball' Game on Vioxx Questions: Lawyer." Matt Daily. *Reuters*, July 18, 2005.

"Merck Vioxx By-the-Numbers." *Wall Street Journal*, November 9, 2007.

"Mile Trivia." Mike Tymn. *Running Times Magazine*, May 2004.

"Mind Your Omega-3's." Karlene Karst. *Health N Vitality Magazine*, January 2003.

"Mortality and Life Expectancy in Relation to Long-term Cigarette, Cigar and Pipe Smoking." The Zutphen Study. 2007.

"Nexium Acid Reflux Drug Approved for Children Ages 1–11." *Fox News*, February 28, 2008.

"Outcry over Pets in Pet Food." *Los Angeles Times,* January 6, 2002.

"Pesticides Build Up in Our Bodies." Update, Spring 2004. www.panna.org/docsTrespass/chemicalTrespass2004.dv.html.

"Pesticides in the Environment." Pesticide fact sheets and tutorial, module 6. www.cornell.edu.

"Power Steer." Michael Pollan. *New York Times*, March 31, 2002.

"The Purple Pill." Christine Bittaro. *BrandWeek*, October 11, 2004.

"Rethinking the Meat-Guzzler." Mark Bittman. *New York Times*, January 27, 2008.

"A Review of the Welfare Issues for Sows and Piglets in Relation to Housing." J. L. Barnett et al. *Australian Journal of Agricultural Research* 52, 2001, 1–28.

"Scientists: Factory Farming Drop Could End Mad Cow." *CNN/Reuters*, December 4, 2000.

"Scientists Finding Out What Losing Sleep Does to a Body." Rob Stein. *Washington Post Sunday*, October 9, 2005.

"A Search for Answers in Russert's Death." Denise Grady. *New York Times*, June 17, 2008.

"Self-diagnosis from TV Drug Ads Can Be Dangerous." Bill Hendrick. *Atlanta Journal-Constitution*, January 8, 2008.

"Settling Doubts about Livestock Stress." Don Comis. *Agricultural Research*, March 2005.

"Sleep Drugs Found Only Mildly Effective but Wildly Popular." Stephanie Saul. *New York Times*, October 23, 2007.

"Sleeping Pills For Kids?" 2007 International Bad Product Awards. Consumerist.com.

"Stress a Major Health Problem in the U.S." American Psychological Association. October 24, 2007.

"Sugar Consumption 'Off the Charts' Say Health Experts: HHS/USDA Urged to Commission Review of Sugar's Health Impact." CSPI, December 30, 1998. www.cspinet.org/new/sugar.htm.

"Supreme Court Rules on Artificially Colored Farm Raised Salmon." Jim Porter. *Law Review*, April 4, 2008.

"Sweeping Changes to British Farming." *BBC News*, December 1, 1965.

"These 10 Top Nutritional Performers Can Transform Your Diet—and Possibly Your Life." Carol Ness. *San Francisco Chronicle*, January 4, 2006.

"The Truth about Organic Foods." Jessica DeCostole. *Redbook*, September 2007.

"Unhappiness Has Risen in the Past Decade." Sharon Jayson. *USA Today*, January 8, 2006.

"Vioxx Risk Cited Scientist in 1998: Firm Downplayed Safety Concerns, Lawyer Contends." *Bloomberg News*, 2005.

"Vioxx Risks Understated, According to Trial Evidence." Alex Berenson. *New York Times*, July 21, 2005.

"The Welfare of Sows in Gestation Crates: A Summary of the Scientific Evidence." *Farm Sanctuary*, 1995.

"Why the Organic Revolution Had to Happen." John Simpson. *The Observer*, April 21, 2001.

"Your Body Is Younger Than You Think." Nicholas Wade. *New York Times*, 2005.

"Your Body's Many Cries for Water." Fereydoon Batmanghelidj. Global Health Solutions, Vienne, VA, 1995.

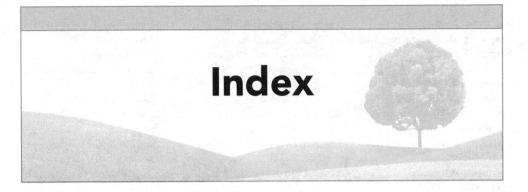

Index

Page numbers in *italics* refer to illustrations.

treatment:
  before-the-fact vs. after-the-fact, 18
  myths about, 22
truth, 6, 66, 144
tryptophan, 138
Tufts University, 79
turnip greens, 72
Twinkies, 9

UltraPrevention (Hyman), 49, 85
unconscious competence, 6
unconscious incompetence, 6
uniqueness, 141, *142*
United Nations, 50
United States:
  DDT ban in, 53
  as "fast food nation," 10
unsaturated fats, *see* fish fats
urine:
  color of, 115
  drugs in, 110–11

valerian, 138
vegetables, 10, 39, 72–75, 81, 83–84, 89, 92–93, 119
  dark, green, leafy, 79
  pesticides in, 53, 54
  raw, 91, 103
  root, 93
  steamed, 91, 103

variety of, 93
  see also specific vegetables
Vioxx, 32–34
viruses, 65–67, 71, 75, 81
vitamin D3, 97–98
vitamins, 97–98
Voltaire, 23

Waitley, Denis, 125
walking, 117
Ward, Artemus, 1
Washington, University of, 54
water, 69, 75, 85, 87, 109–16
  acidity of, 112
  amount of, 113, 114, 115
  best source of, 111
  drugs in, 110–11
  filtered, 112–13
  lymph system and, 113–14, 115
  ten-day plan for, 115
weight loss, 4–5, 114, 158
weight-loss clinics and businesses, 11
weight problems, 47, 116, 137, 159–60
  see also obesity; overweight
Weil, Andrew, 66
wellness, 21
  fitness vs., 11
Wendy's, 86
White, Thomas, 111

White Menaces, 49
white tea, 80
Whole Foods Market, 39, 92, 94, 95, 103, 152
wine, 102–3
witch hazel, 101
women:
  cancer in, 14
  drug testing and, 32
  stress in, 122
Wonder Bread, 8–9, 48
World Health Organization, 17, 29
Worthington, Everett, Jr., 129–32

yoga, 118
Yumi Tea, 80

Zenn, J. Michael (author), 159–63
  appearance of, 7–8, 40
  childhood memories of, 8, 39
  eating habits of, 10
  family background of, 104
  fortieth birthday of, 7, 11–12
  McDonald's job of, 10
  as overweight and without energy, 7–8, 11
  Self-Health Revolution of, 12, 37–40
zeranol, 59